*Quick*FACTS™

Lung
CANCER

What You Need to Know—NOW

SECOND EDITION

*Quick*FACTS™

From the Experts at the American Cancer Society

Lung
CANCER

What You Need to Know—NOW

SECOND EDITION

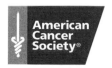

Published by the American Cancer Society/Health Promotions
250 Williams Street NW, Atlanta, Georgia 30303-1002 USA

For permission to reprint any materials from this publication, contact the publisher at **permissionrequest@cancer.org.**

Printed in the United States of America
Cover designed by Jill Dible, Atlanta, GA
Composition by Graphic Composition, Inc., Bogart, GA

5 4 3 2 1   13 14 15 16 17

Library of Congress Cataloging-in-Publication Data

Quick facts lung cancer : what you need to know—now / from the Experts at the American Cancer Society.—2nd ed.
     p. cm.—(Quick facts)
    Includes bibliographical references and index.
    ISBN 978-1-60443-061-5 (pbk. : alk. paper)—
    ISBN 1-60443-061-3 (pbk. : alk. paper)
    1. Lungs—Cancer—Popular works. I. American Cancer Society.
RC280.L8Q53 2013
616.99′424—dc23

                              2011021710

Quantity discounts on bulk purchases of this book are available. Book excerpts can also be created to fit specific needs. For information, please contact the American Cancer Society, Health Promotions Publishing, 250 Williams Street NW, Atlanta, GA 30303-1002, or send an e-mail to—**trade.sales@cancer.org.**

A Note to the Reader

This information represents the views of the doctors and nurses serving on the American Cancer Society's Cancer Information Database Editorial Board. These views are based on their interpretation of studies published in medical journals, as well as their own professional experience.

The treatment information in this book is not official policy of the Society and is not intended as medical advice to replace the expertise and judgment of your cancer care team. It is intended to help you and your family make informed decisions, together with your doctor.

Your doctor may have reasons for suggesting a treatment plan different from these general treatment options. Don't hesitate to ask him or her questions about your treatment options.

For more information, contact your American Cancer Society at **800-227-2345** or **cancer.org**.

TABLE OF CONTENTS

Diagnosis and Staging

Treatment

Resources

Your Lung Cancer

What Is Cancer?

The body is made up of trillions of living cells. Normal body cells grow, divide, and die in an orderly fashion. During the early years of a person's life, normal cells divide faster to allow the person to grow. After the person becomes an adult, most cells divide only to replace worn-out or dying cells or to repair injuries.

Cancer begins when **cells** in a part of the body start to grow out of control. There are many kinds of cancer, but they all start because of out-of-control growth of abnormal cells. Cancer cell growth is different from normal cell growth. Instead of dying, cancer cells continue to grow and form new, abnormal cells. Cancer cells can also invade (grow into) other tissues, something that normal cells cannot do. Growing out of control and invading other tissues are what makes a cell a cancer cell.

Cells become cancer cells because of damage to **DNA**. DNA is in every cell and directs all its

*Terms in **bold type** are further explained in the glossary, beginning on page 169.

actions. In a normal cell, when DNA becomes damaged, the cell either repairs the damage or the cell dies. In cancer cells, the damaged DNA is not repaired, but the cell doesn't die like it should. Instead, this cell goes on making new cells that the body does not need. These new cells will all have the same damaged DNA as the first cell.

People can inherit damaged DNA, but most DNA damage is caused by mistakes that happen while the normal cell is reproducing or by something in our environment. Sometimes the cause of the DNA damage is something obvious, such as cigarette smoking. But often no clear cause is found.

In most cases, the cancer cells form a **tumor**. Some cancers, like leukemia, rarely form tumors. Instead, these cancer cells involve the blood and blood-forming organs and circulate through other tissues where they grow.

Cancer cells often travel to other parts of the body, where they begin to grow and form new tumors that replace normal **tissue**. This process is called **metastasis**. It happens when the cancer cells get into the bloodstream or lymph vessels of the body.

No matter where a cancer spreads, it is always named for the place where it started. For example, breast cancer that has spread to the liver is still called breast cancer, not liver cancer. Likewise, prostate cancer that has spread to the bone is metastatic prostate cancer, not bone cancer.

Different types of cancer can behave very differently. For example, lung cancer and breast cancer are very different diseases. They grow at different rates and respond to different treatments. That is why people with cancer need treatment that is aimed at their particular kind of cancer.

Not all tumors are cancerous. Tumors that aren't cancerous are called **benign**. A **benign tumor** can cause problems—it can grow very large and press on healthy organs and tissues. But benign tumors cannot invade other tissues. Because they can't invade, they also can't spread to other parts of the body (**metastasize**). These tumors are almost never life threatening.

What Is Lung Cancer?

Lung cancer is a cancer that starts in the lungs. To understand lung cancer, it helps to know about the normal structure and function of the lungs.

The Lungs

Your lungs are 2 sponge-like organs found in your chest. Your right lung is divided into 3 sections, called **lobes**. Your left lung has 2 lobes. The left lung is smaller because the heart takes up more room on that side of the body.

When you breathe in, air enters through your mouth or nose and goes into your lungs through the **trachea** (windpipe). The trachea divides into tubes called the **bronchi** (or **bronchus**, in the singular), which divide into smaller branches called

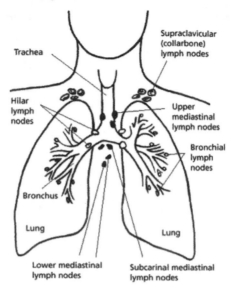

bronchioles. At the end of the bronchioles are tiny air sacs known as **alveoli**. Many tiny blood vessels run through the alveoli. They absorb oxygen from the inhaled air into your bloodstream and pass carbon dioxide from the body into the alveoli. The carbon dioxide is expelled from the body when you exhale. Taking in oxygen and getting rid of carbon dioxide are your lungs' main functions.

A thin lining, called the **pleura,** surrounds the lungs. The pleura protects your lungs and helps them slide back and forth against the chest wall as they expand and contract during breathing. Below the lungs, a dome-shaped muscle called the **diaphragm** separates the chest from the abdomen.

When you breathe, the diaphragm moves up and down, forcing air in and out of the lungs.

The Start and Spread of Lung Cancer

Lung cancers can start in the cells lining the bronchi and in other parts of the lung, such as the bronchioles or alveoli. Lung cancers are thought to start as areas of **precancerous** changes in the lung. The first changes happen in the **genes** of the cells themselves and may cause the cells to grow faster. The cells may look a bit abnormal if examined under a microscope, but at this point, they do not form a mass or tumor. They cannot be seen on an **x-ray** and they do not cause **symptoms**.

Over time, these precancerous changes in the cells may progress to true cancer. As a cancer develops, the cancer cells may produce chemicals that cause new blood vessels to form nearby. These new blood vessels nourish the cancer cells, which can continue to grow and form a tumor large enough to be seen on imaging tests such as x-rays.

At some point, cells from the cancer may break away from the original tumor and spread to other parts of the body. As noted earlier, this process is called metastasis. Lung cancer is often a life-threatening disease because it tends to spread even before it can be detected on an imaging test, such as a chest x-ray.

The Lymphatic System

One of the ways cancer can spread is through the **lymphatic system**. The lymphatic system has several parts. **Lymph nodes** are small, bean-shaped collections of **immune system** cells (cells that fight infection) that are connected by lymphatic vessels. Lymphatic vessels are similar to small veins but carry a clear fluid called **lymph** instead of blood. Lymph contains excess fluid and waste products from body tissues, as well as immune system cells.

Lung cancer cells can enter lymphatic vessels and begin to grow in lymph nodes around the bronchi and in the **mediastinum** (the area between the 2 lungs). When lung cancer cells have reached the lymph nodes, they are more likely to have spread to other organs of the body as well. The **stage** (extent) of the cancer and decisions about treatment are based on whether the cancer has spread to certain groups of lymph nodes. These topics are discussed on pages 54–67 in the section "How Is Lung Cancer Staged?"

Types of Lung Cancer

There are 2 major types of lung cancer:

- non–small cell lung cancer (NSCLC)
- small cell lung cancer (SCLC)

If a lung cancer has characteristics of both types, it is called a mixed small cell/large cell cancer. This is uncommon.

These 2 types of lung cancer are treated very differently. This book includes information about both types.

Non–Small Cell Lung Cancer

About 85% to 90% of lung cancers are **non–small cell lung cancer (NSCLC)**. There are 3 main subtypes of NSCLC. The cells in these subtypes differ in size, shape, and chemical make-up when looked at under a microscope. These subtypes are grouped together because the approach to their treatment and **prognosis** (outlook) are very similar.

Squamous cell (epidermoid) carcinoma

About 25% to 30% of all lung cancers are **squamous cell carcinomas**. These cancers start in early versions of squamous cells, which are flat cells that line the inside of the airways in the lungs. They are often linked to a history of smoking and tend to be found in the middle of the lungs, near a bronchus.

Adenocarcinoma

About 40% of lung cancers are **adenocarcinomas**. These cancers start in early versions of cells that would normally secrete such substances as mucus. This type of lung cancer occurs mainly in people who smoke or have smoked, but it is also the most common type of lung cancer seen in nonsmokers. It is more common in women than in men, and it is more likely than other types of lung cancer to occur in younger people.

Adenocarcinoma is usually found in the outer region of the lung. It tends to grow more slowly than other types of lung cancer, and it is more likely to be found before it has spread outside the lung. People with a type of adenocarcinoma called adenocarcinoma in situ (previously called bronchioloalveolar carcinoma) tend to have a better prognosis than those with other types of lung cancer.

Large cell (undifferentiated) carcinoma

Large-cell undifferentiated carcinoma accounts for about 10% to 15% of lung cancers. It may appear in any part of the lung. It tends to grow and spread quickly, which can make it harder to treat. Large cell neuroendocrine carcinoma, a subtype of large cell carcinoma, is a fast-growing cancer that is very similar to small cell lung cancer.

Other subtypes

There are a few other subtypes of non–small cell lung cancer, such as adenosquamous carcinoma and sarcomatoid carcinoma. These subtypes are much less common.

Small Cell Lung Cancer

About 10% to 15% of all lung cancers are **small cell lung cancer (SCLC)**, named for the size of the cancer cells when seen under a microscope. Other names for SCLC are oat cell cancer, oat cell carcinoma, and small cell undifferentiated carcinoma. It is very rare for someone who has never smoked to have small cell lung cancer.

SCLC often starts in the bronchi near the center of the chest, and it tends to spread widely through the body fairly early in the course of the disease, usually before it causes symptoms. The cancer cells can multiply quickly, form large tumors, and spread to lymph nodes and other organs, such as the bones, brain, adrenal glands, and liver. Because the cancer cells multiply and spread quickly, surgery is rarely an option and never the only treatment recommended. Chemotherapy, which can reach cancer cells anywhere in the body, is an important part of treatment for all small cell lung cancers, as long as a person is healthy enough to tolerate it.

Other Types of Lung Cancer

In addition to the 2 main types of lung cancer, other tumors can occur in the lungs. **Carcinoid tumors** of the lung account for fewer than 5% of lung tumors. Most are slow-growing tumors that are called typical carcinoid tumors. They are generally cured by surgery. Some typical carcinoid tumors can spread, but they usually have a better prognosis than small cell or non–small cell lung cancers. Less common are **atypical** carcinoid tumors. The prognosis for these tumors is somewhere between typical carcinoids and small cell lung cancer. For more information about typical and atypical carcinoid tumors, call the American Cancer Society at **800-227-2345** and request the document *Lung Carcinoid Tumor* or visit **cancer.org**.

There are other, even more rare, lung tumors such as adenoid cystic carcinomas, hamartomas, lymphomas, and sarcomas. These tumors are treated differently from the more common types of lung cancer.

Cancers that start in other organs (such as the breast, pancreas, kidney, or skin) can sometimes metastasize to the lungs, but these cancers are not considered lung cancers. For example, cancer that starts in the breast and spreads to the lungs is still called breast cancer, not lung cancer. Treatment for **metastatic cancer** to the lungs depends on where the cancer started (the **primary site**).

What Are the Key Statistics About Lung Cancer?

Most lung cancer statistics include both small cell and non–small cell lung cancers.

Not counting skin cancer, lung cancer is the second most common cancer in men (after prostate cancer) and women (after breast cancer). It accounts for about 14% of all new cancer diagnoses. The American Cancer Society's most recent estimates for lung cancer in the United States are for 2012:

- In 2012, about 226,160 new cases of lung cancer will be diagnosed (116,470 among men and 109,690 among women).
- In 2012, there will be an estimated 160,340 deaths from lung cancer (87,750 among men and 72,590 among women), accounting for about 28% of all cancer deaths.

Lung cancer is by far the leading cause of cancer death among both men and women. Each year more people die of lung cancer than of colon, breast, and prostate cancers combined. Lung cancer mainly occurs in older people. About 2 out of 3 people with lung cancer are older than 65; fewer than 2% of all cases are found in people younger than 45. The average age at the time of **diagnosis** is about 71.

Overall, the chance that a man will have lung cancer in his lifetime is about 1 in 13; for a woman, the risk is about 1 in 16. These numbers include both smokers and nonsmokers. The risk is much higher for smokers. Black men are about 40% more likely to have lung cancer than white men. The rate is about the same in black women and white women. Both black and white women have lower rates than men, but that gap is closing. The rate of lung cancer has been dropping among men for many years and is just beginning to drop in women after a long period of rising.

Statistics on survival in people with lung cancer vary depending on the cancer's stage at diagnosis. Survival statistics based on the stage of the cancer are discussed on pages 68–70. Despite the very serious prognosis of lung cancer, some people are cured. More than 350,000 people alive today have received a diagnosis of lung cancer at some point.

Risk Factors and Causes

What Are the Risk Factors for Lung Cancer?

A **risk factor** is anything that affects a person's chance of getting a disease such as cancer. Different cancers have different risk factors. For example, unprotected exposure to strong sunlight is a risk factor for skin cancer. Risk factors don't tell us everything. Having a risk factor, or even several risk factors, does not mean that you will get the disease. And some people who get the disease may not have any known risk factors. Even if a person with lung cancer has a risk factor, it is difficult to know how much that risk factor may have contributed to the cancer's development.

Several risk factors can make it more likely you will get lung cancer.

Factors Known to Affect Lung Cancer Risk

Tobacco smoke

Smoking is by far the leading risk factor for lung cancer. In the early part of the 20th century, lung cancer was much less common than other types of cancer. Rates of lung cancer increased once manufactured cigarettes became readily available and more people began smoking.

About 80% of lung cancer deaths are thought to result from smoking. The risk of lung cancer among smokers is many times higher than that of nonsmokers. The longer you smoke and the more packs per day you smoke, the greater your risk. The percentage of lung cancer deaths that result from smoking is probably higher for small cell lung cancer.

Cigar smoking and pipe smoking are almost as likely to cause lung cancer as cigarette smoking. Smoking low-tar or "light" cigarettes increases lung cancer risk as much as regular cigarettes. There is concern that menthol cigarettes may increase the risk even more, as the menthol may allow smokers to inhale more deeply.

If you stop smoking before cancer develops, your damaged lung tissue will gradually start to repair itself. No matter what your age or how long you've smoked, quitting may lower your risk of lung cancer and help you live longer. People who stop smoking before age 50 cut in half their risk of dying in the next 15 years as compared with those who continue to smoke. For help quitting, call the American Cancer Society at **800-227-2345** and ask for the *Guide to Quitting Smoking* or visit our Web site, **cancer.org**.

Secondhand smoke: If you don't smoke, breathing in the smoke of others (called **secondhand smoke** or environmental tobacco smoke) can increase your risk of lung cancer. A nonsmoker who lives with a smoker has about a 20% to 30% greater risk of lung cancer than one who lives with a non-smoker. People who have been exposed to tobacco smoke in the workplace are also more likely to get lung cancer. Secondhand smoke is thought to cause more than 3,000 deaths from lung cancer each year.

Some evidence suggests that certain people are more susceptible to the cancer-causing effect of tobacco smoke than others.

Radon

Radon is a naturally occurring radioactive gas that results from the breakdown of uranium in soil and rocks. It cannot be seen, tasted, or smelled. According to the U.S. Environmental Protection Agency (EPA), radon is the second leading cause of lung cancer and the leading cause among non-smokers in the United States.

Outdoors, there is so little radon that it is not likely to be dangerous. But indoors, radon can be more concentrated. When radon is breathed in, it enters the lungs and exposes them to small amounts of radiation. This exposure may increase a person's risk of lung cancer. Houses built on soil with natural uranium deposits can have high indoor radon levels, particularly in basements. Studies have found that the risk of lung cancer is higher in those who have lived for many years in a radon-contaminated house. The lung cancer risk from radon is much lower than that from tobacco smoke. However, the risk from radon is much higher in people who smoke than in those who don't.

Radon levels in the soil vary across the country, but they can be high almost anywhere. If you are concerned about radon exposure, you can use a radon detection kit to test the levels in your home. State and local offices of the EPA can also give you the names of reliable companies that can test for radon and help you fix the problem, if needed. For more information on radon, visit the American Cancer Society Web site at **cancer.org** or call **800-227-2345**.

Asbestos

Workplace exposure to asbestos fibers is an important risk factor for lung cancer. Studies have found that people who work with asbestos (in some mines, mills, textile plants, places where insulation is used, shipyards, etc.) are several times more likely to die of lung cancer. In workers exposed to asbestos who also smoke, the lung cancer risk is much greater than even adding the risks from these exposures separately. It's not clear to what extent low-level or short-term exposure to asbestos might raise lung cancer risk.

In recent years, government regulations have greatly reduced the use of asbestos in commercial and industrial products. It is still present in many homes and older buildings, but it is not usually considered harmful as long as it is not released into the air by deterioration, demolition, or renovation.

Both smokers and nonsmokers exposed to asbestos also have a greater risk of **mesothelioma**, a type of cancer that starts in the pleura. Mesothelioma is not usually considered a type of lung cancer. For more information on malignant mesothelioma or asbestos, visit the American Cancer Society Web site, **cancer.org**, or call **800-227-2345**.

Other cancer-causing agents in the workplace

There are other **carcinogens** (cancer-causing agents) found in some workplaces that can increase lung cancer risk:

- radioactive ores, such as uranium
- inhaled chemicals or minerals, such as arsenic, beryllium, cadmium, silica, vinyl chloride, nickel compounds, chromium compounds, coal products, mustard gas, and chloromethyl ethers
- diesel exhaust

The government and industry have taken steps in recent years to help protect workers from many of these exposures. But the dangers are still present, and if you work around these agents, you should be careful to limit your exposure whenever possible.

Radiation therapy to the lungs

People who have had radiation therapy to the chest for other cancers are at higher risk for lung cancer, particularly if they smoke. Typical patients are those treated for **Hodgkin disease** or women who receive radiation to the chest after a mastectomy for breast cancer. Women who receive radiation therapy to the breast after a lumpectomy do not appear to have a higher than expected risk of lung cancer.

Arsenic

High levels of arsenic in drinking water may increase the risk of lung cancer. This risk is even more pronounced in smokers.

Personal or family history of lung cancer

If you have had lung cancer, you are at higher risk for another lung cancer. Siblings and children of those who have had lung cancer may have a slightly higher risk of lung cancer themselves, especially if the relative received the diagnosis at a younger age. It is not clear how much this risk might be due to genetics and how much might be from shared household exposures (such as tobacco smoke or radon).

Researchers have found that genetics does seem to play a role in some families with a strong history of lung cancer. For example, people who inherit certain DNA changes in a particular **chromosome** (chromosome 6) are at higher risk for lung cancer, even if they smoke only a little. Currently, there is no way to routinely test for these inherited DNA changes. Research is ongoing in this area.

Certain dietary supplements

Studies looking at the possible role of anti-oxidant supplements in reducing lung cancer risk have not been promising so far. In fact, 2 large studies found that smokers who took beta carotene supplements actually were at *increased* risk for lung cancer. The results of these studies suggest that smokers should avoid taking beta carotene supplements.

Air pollution

Air pollution (especially from heavily trafficked roads) appears to raise the risk of lung cancer slightly. This risk is far less than the risk caused by smoking, but some researchers estimate that about 5% of all deaths from lung cancer worldwide may be due to outdoor air pollution.

Factors with Uncertain or Unproven Effects on Lung Cancer Risk

Marijuana

There are some reasons to think that marijuana smoking might increase lung cancer risk. Many of the cancer-causing substances in tobacco are also found in marijuana. Marijuana also contains more tar than cigarettes. Tar is the sticky, solid material that remains after burning, and it is thought to contain most of the harmful substances in smoke. Marijuana cigarettes (joints) are typically smoked all the way to the end, where tar content is the highest. Marijuana is also inhaled very deeply and the smoke is held in the lungs for a long time. In addition, because marijuana is an illegal substance, it is not possible to control what other substances it might contain.

In a given day or week, however, those who use marijuana tend to smoke fewer marijuana cigarettes than those who smoke tobacco cigarettes. For example, a light smoker may smoke half a pack of cigarettes a day (10 cigarettes), but 10 marijuana cigarettes in a day would be very heavy use of marijuana. In one study, most people who smoked marijuana did so 2 to 3 times per month. The lesser amount smoked would make it harder to see an impact on lung cancer risk.

It has been hard to study whether there is a link between marijuana and lung cancer because it is not easy to gather information about the use of illegal drugs. Many marijuana smokers also smoke cigarettes, making it hard to know how much of the risk is from tobacco and how much is from marijuana. In the very limited studies done so far, marijuana use has not been strongly linked to lung cancer, but more research in this area is needed.

Talc and talcum powder

Talc is a mineral that, in its natural form, may contain asbestos. In the past, some studies suggested that talc miners and millers have a higher risk of lung cancer and other respiratory diseases because of exposure to industrial grade talc. Recent studies of talc miners have not found an increase in lung cancer rate.

Talcum powder is made from talc. By law since 1973, all home-use talcum products (baby, body, and facial powders) in the United States have been asbestos-free. The use of cosmetic talcum powder has not been found to increase the risk of lung cancer.

Do We Know What Causes Lung Cancer?

Smoking

Tobacco smoking is by far the leading cause of both non–small cell and small cell lung cancer.

About 80% of lung cancer deaths are caused directly by smoking, and that percentage is probably higher for small cell lung cancer. Most small cell lung cancers are caused by smoking, although some are not.

Lung Cancer in Nonsmokers

Not all people who get lung cancer are smokers. Many people with lung cancer are former smokers, but many others never smoked at all. Some of the causes for lung cancer in nonsmokers include exposure to radon, which accounts for about 20,000 cases of lung cancer each year, and exposure to secondhand smoke. Workplace exposure to asbestos, diesel exhaust, or certain other chemicals can also cause lung cancer in nonsmokers. A small portion of lung cancers occur in people with no known risk factors for the disease, so there must be other factors that we do not yet know about.

Genetic factors seem to play a role in at least some of these cancers. Lung cancers in nonsmokers are often different in some ways from those that occur in smokers. They tend to occur at a younger age, often affecting people in their 30s or 40s (whereas in smokers, the average age at diagnosis is over 70). The cancers that occur in nonsmokers often have gene **mutations** that are different from those seen in the tumors of smokers. In some cases, these gene mutations can be used to guide decisions about therapy.

Gene Changes that May Lead to Lung Cancer

Scientists have begun to understand how the known risk factors for lung cancer may change the DNA of cells in the lungs, causing them to grow abnormally and form cancers. DNA is the chemical in each of our cells that makes up our genes—the instructions for how our cells function. We usually look like our parents because they are the source of our DNA. However, DNA affects more than how we look. It also can influence our risk for certain diseases, such as some kinds of cancer.

Some genes contain instructions for controlling when cells grow and divide. Genes that promote cell division are called **oncogenes**. Genes that slow down cell division or cause cells to die at the right time are called **tumor suppressor genes**. Cancer can be caused by DNA changes that turn on oncogenes or turn off tumor suppressor genes.

Inherited gene changes

Some people inherit DNA mutations that greatly increase their risk for certain types of cancer. However, inherited mutations are not thought to cause many lung cancers. Still, genes do seem to play a role in some families with a history of lung cancer. For example, some people seem to inherit a reduced ability to break down certain types of cancer-causing chemicals in the body, such as those found in tobacco smoke. This trait could put them at higher risk for lung cancer.

Other people may inherit faulty **DNA repair** mechanisms, making it more likely they will end up with DNA mutations. Every time a cell prepares to divide into 2 new cells, it must duplicate its DNA. This process is not perfect, and copying errors sometimes occur. Cells normally have repair enzymes that proofread the DNA to help prevent these errors. People with repair enzymes that don't work as well might be especially vulnerable to cancer-causing chemicals and radiation. Researchers are developing tests to help identify such people, but these tests are not yet reliable enough for routine use. For now, doctors recommend that all people avoid tobacco smoke and other exposures that could increase their cancer risk.

Acquired gene changes

Gene changes related to lung cancer are usually acquired during life, not inherited. Acquired mutations in lung cells often result from exposure to environmental factors, such as cancer-causing chemicals in tobacco smoke. Some gene changes, however, may just be random events that happen inside a cell without an external cause.

Acquired changes in certain genes, such as the *TP53* or *p16* tumor suppressor genes and the *KRAS* oncogene, are thought to be important in the development of lung cancer. Changes in these and other genes may also make some lung cancers more likely to grow and spread rapidly. Not all lung cancers share the same gene mutations. Undoubtedly, there are other gene mutations that have not yet been discovered, which could affect lung cancer development.

Prevention and Detection

Can Lung Cancer Be Prevented?

Not all cases of lung cancer can be prevented, but there are some ways you can reduce lung cancer risk. The best way to reduce your risk of lung cancer is to abstain from smoking and to avoid breathing in other people's smoke. If you would like help quitting smoking, call the American Cancer Society at **800-227-2345** or visit our Web site at **cancer.org** and see our *Guide to Quitting Smoking*.

Radon is an important cause of lung cancer. You can reduce your exposure to radon by having your home tested and, if needed, treated. Avoiding exposure to known cancer-causing chemicals in the workplace and elsewhere may also be helpful (see the section on risk factors in the previous chapter). People working where these exposures are common should try to minimize exposure.

A healthy diet with lots of fruits and vegetables may also help reduce your risk of lung cancer. Some evidence suggests that a diet high in fruits and vegetables may help protect against lung cancer in both smokers and nonsmokers. Any positive effect of fruits and vegetables on lung cancer risk would be much less than the increased risk from smoking.

Attempts to reduce the risk of lung cancer in current or former smokers by giving them high doses of vitamins or vitamin-like drugs have not been successful. Some studies have found that beta carotene, a nutrient related to vitamin A, appears to increase the rate of lung cancer in these people.

Some people with lung cancer do not have any apparent risk factors. Although we know how to prevent most lung cancers, at this time we don't know how to prevent all of them.

Can Lung Cancer Be Found Early?

It is often hard to find lung cancer early. Symptoms of lung cancer usually do not appear until the disease is already advanced. Even when symptoms of lung cancer do appear, many people mistake them for other problems, such as an infection or the long-term effects of smoking, which can delay diagnosis even further.

Some lung cancers are diagnosed early because they are found as a result of tests for other conditions. Lung cancer can be found by **imaging tests** (such as a chest x-ray or **CT scan**), **bronchoscopy**, or **sputum cytology** done for other reasons in patients with heart disease, pneumonia, or other lung conditions.

Screening for Lung Cancer

Screening is the use of tests or examinations to detect a disease in people with no symptoms of that disease. For example, the Pap test is used as a screening test for cervical cancer. Because lung cancer usually spreads beyond the lungs before causing any symptoms, an effective screening test for lung cancer could save many lives.

Until recently, no lung cancer screening test had been shown to lower the risk of dying of this disease. Earlier studies of 2 possible screening tests—chest x ray and sputum cytology—did not find that these tests could detect lung cancers early enough to improve the chance for cure. For this reason, major medical organizations have not recommended routine screening with these tests for the general public or even for people at increased risk, such as smokers.

Low-dose spiral CT

A newer type of CT scan, known as low-dose **spiral CT** (or helical CT) has shown some promise in detecting lung cancer early in heavy smokers and former smokers. Spiral CT of the chest provides more detailed pictures than a chest x-ray and is better at finding small abnormalities in the lungs. The type of CT scan used for lung cancer screening uses less radiation than a standard chest x-ray. It also does not require the use of an intravenous (IV) contrast dye.

In the National Lung Screening Trial (NLST), spiral CT scans were compared with chest x-rays in people at high risk for lung cancer to see whether spiral CTs could lower the risk of death of lung cancer. The study included more than 50,000 current or former smokers aged 55 to 74. Participants had at least a 30 pack-year history of smoking (equivalent to smoking a pack a day for 30 years or 2 packs a day for 15 years). Former smokers must have quit within the past 15 years. People were not eligible for the study if they had a prior history of lung cancer or lung cancer symptoms, or if they needed to use oxygen at home to help them breathe. All participants received either 3 spiral CT scans or 3 chest x-rays, each a year apart. They were then observed for several years.

The study found that people who received spiral CT scans had a 20% lower chance of dying of lung cancer than those who received chest x-rays. They were also 7% less likely to die of any cause, although the exact reasons for this are not yet clear.

Researchers are now analyzing the full results of the study, and there are some questions yet to be answered. For example, it is not clear whether screening with spiral CT scans would have the same effect on different groups of people, such as those who smoked less (or not at all) or people younger than age 55. The lung cancers that were found early in this study were non–small cell lung cancers. At this time, it is not clear whether low-dose spiral CT is effective for early detection of small cell lung cancers. The best screening schedule—how often scans should be done, how long they should be continued, etc.—is also unclear.

A spiral CT scan is also known to have some disadvantages. This test can find other abnormalities that are not cancer but require further investigation, sometimes leading to unnecessary tests or procedures in some people. (About 1 in 4 people in the NLST had such a finding.) This may include more CT scans or more invasive procedures, such as needle biopsies or surgery. A very small number of people who did not have cancer (or had a very early stage) have died as a result of these procedures. Each spiral CT scan also exposes the recipient to a small amount of radiation—less than a standard CT scan but more than a chest x-ray. This exposure increases a person's risk of breast, lung, and thyroid cancers later on. The advantages and disadvantages of spiral CT scanning should be discussed if you and your doctor are considering whether this test is right for you.

Current Screening Recommendations

Although the American Cancer Society has not yet developed lung cancer screening guidelines, it plans to do so in the future. In the meantime, some people who are at higher risk (and their doctors) may consider whether screening is appropriate for them.

While a full cancer screening guideline is being developed, the American Cancer Society has created interim guidance for people and their doctors regarding the use of low-dose CT scans for the early detection of lung cancer:

- People between the ages of 55 and 74 who meet the entry criteria of the NLST (see page 28) and are concerned about their risk of lung cancer may consider screening for lung cancer. With their doctor, people interested in screening should weigh the known benefits of screening with its known limits and risks in order to make a shared decision about screening.

- Doctors may choose to discuss lung cancer screening with their patients who meet NLST entry criteria.

- For people who do not meet the NLST entry criteria (because of age, smoking history, etc.), it is not clear whether the possible benefits of screening outweigh the harms, so screening in these people is not recommended at this time. The recommendation not to screen applies in particular to people with no smoking history, for whom the screening is more likely to cause possible harms than benefits. Whether to screen people whose age or smoking history would have made them ineligible for the NLST will be addressed during the guidelines development process as more data become available.

- People who choose to be screened should follow the NLST protocol for annual screening. Screening should be done through an organized screening program at an institution with expertise in spiral CT screening and with access to a multidisciplinary team skilled in finding and treating abnormal lung lesions. Referring doctors should help their patients find institutions with this expertise.

- There is always benefit to quitting smoking. Active smokers entering a lung screening program should be urged to enter a smoking cessation program. Screening should not be viewed as an alternative to quitting smoking.

- For people considering screening (and their doctors), some statistics from the NLST may be helpful. Of the nearly 26,000 people screened by low-dose CT in the NLST, 1,060 received a diagnosis of lung cancer. Screening is estimated to have prevented 88 lung cancer deaths and caused 16 deaths. Of the 16 deaths, 6 were in patients who ultimately were found not to have cancer.

For more detailed information on the interim guidance, please call the American Cancer Society at **800-227-2345** and request the document *American Cancer Society Interim Guidance on Lung Cancer Screening* or visit **cancer.org**.

Even with the promising results from the NLST, people who are current smokers should realize that the best way to avoid dying of lung cancer is to stop smoking. For help quitting smoking, call the American Cancer Society at **800-227-2345** or visit **cancer.org**.

Diagnosis and Staging

How Is Lung Cancer Diagnosed?

Most lung cancers are not found until they start to cause symptoms. Symptoms can suggest that a person has lung cancer, but the actual diagnosis is made by examining lung cells under a microscope.

Common Signs and Symptoms of Lung Cancer

Although most lung cancers do not cause any symptoms until they have spread too far to be cured, symptoms do occur in some people with early lung cancer. If you go to your doctor when you first notice symptoms, your cancer might be diagnosed at an earlier stage when treatment is more likely to be effective. These are the most common symptoms of lung cancer:

- a cough that does not go away or that gets worse
- chest pain that is often worse with deep breathing, coughing, or laughing
- hoarseness
- weight loss and loss of appetite

- coughing up blood or rust-colored sputum (spit or phlegm)
- shortness of breath
- feeling tired or weak
- recurring infections such as bronchitis and pneumonia
- new onset of wheezing

When lung cancer spreads to distant organs, it can cause a number of symptoms:

- bone pain (in the back or hips)
- neurologic changes (such as headache, weakness or numbness of a limb, dizziness, balance problems, or seizures)
- jaundice (yellowing of the skin and eyes)
- lumps near the surface of the body due to cancer spreading to the skin or to lymph nodes in the neck or above the collarbone

Most of the symptoms listed above are more likely to be caused by conditions other than lung cancer. Still, if you have any of these problems, it is important to see your doctor right away so the cause can be found and treated.

Some lung cancers can cause a group of very specific symptoms. These are often described as syndromes.

Horner syndrome

Cancers of the upper part of the lungs may damage a nerve that passes from the upper chest into your neck, which can cause severe shoulder pain. Doctors sometimes call these Pancoast tumors.

Sometimes these tumors also cause a group of symptoms called Horner syndrome:

- drooping or weakness of one eyelid
- a smaller pupil (dark part in the center of the eye) in the same eye
- reduced or absent sweating on the same side of the face

Conditions other than lung cancer can also cause Horner syndrome.

Superior vena cava syndrome

The superior vena cava (SVC) is a large vein that carries blood from the head and arms back to the heart. It passes next to the upper part of the right lung and the lymph nodes inside the chest. Tumors in this area may push on the SVC, which can cause the blood to back up in the veins. This backup can cause swelling in the face, neck, arms, and upper chest (sometimes with a bluish-red skin color). It can also cause headaches, dizziness, and changes in consciousness if it affects the brain. While SVC syndrome can develop gradually, in some cases it can be life threatening, and it should be treated right away.

Paraneoplastic syndromes

Some lung cancers make hormone-like substances that enter the bloodstream and cause problems with distant tissues and organs, even though the cancer has not spread to those tissues or organs. These problems are called **paraneoplastic syndromes**. Sometimes these syndromes are the first symptoms of lung cancer. Because the symptoms affect other organs, patients and their doctors may first suspect the symptoms are due to a disease other than lung cancer. Non–small cell lung cancer and small cell lung cancer are associated with different paraneoplastic syndromes, so they are described separately below.

Most paraneoplastic syndromes are caused by small cell lung cancer. These are some of the more common paraneoplastic syndromes associated with small cell lung cancer:

Syndrome of inappropriate anti-diuretic hormone (SIADH): In the syndrome of inappropriate anti-diuretic hormone (SIADH), the cancer makes a hormone (ADH) that causes the kidneys to retain water. This water retention causes salt levels in the blood to become very low. Symptoms of SIADH include fatigue, loss of appetite, muscle weakness or cramps, nausea, vomiting, restlessness, and confusion. Without treatment, severe cases of SIADH can lead to seizures and coma.

Cushing syndrome: Cushing syndrome is a disorder that occurs when the body is exposed to high levels of the hormone cortisol. Cushing syndrome can have many causes, but in the case of small cell lung cancer, the lung cancer cells make ACTH, a hormone that causes the adrenal glands to secrete cortisol. Cushing syndrome can lead to such symptoms as weight gain, easy bruising, weakness, drowsiness, fluid retention, high blood pressure, and high blood sugar levels (or even diabetes).

Neurologic problems: Small cell lung cancer can sometimes cause the body's immune system to attack parts of the nervous system, which can lead to problems ranging from muscle weakness to behavioral changes. One example is a muscle disorder called Lambert-Eaton syndrome. This syndrome is characterized by muscle weakness, typically beginning in the muscles around the hips. Symptoms include difficulty chewing, swallowing, or talking; difficulty climbing stairs or getting up from a sitting position; and vision changes, such as blurry vision. A rarer problem is paraneoplastic cerebellar degeneration, which can cause loss of balance, lack of coordination in arm and leg movement, and trouble speaking or swallowing.

Whereas paraneoplastic syndromes are much more common with small cell lung cancer, they can sometimes be caused by non–small cell lung cancer. These are some of the more common paraneoplastic syndromes associated with non–small cell lung cancer:

- high blood calcium levels (**hypercalcemia**), which can cause frequent urination, constipation, nausea, vomiting, weakness, dizziness, confusion, and other nervous system problems
- excess growth of certain bones, especially those in the fingertips, which is often painful
- blood clots
- excess breast growth in men (gynecomastia)

Many of the symptoms above are more likely to be caused by conditions other than lung cancer. If you have any of these problems, see your doctor right away so the cause can be found and treated.

Medical History and Physical Examination

If you have any **signs** or symptoms that suggest you might have lung cancer, your doctor will want to take a medical history to check for risk factors and learn more about your symptoms. Your doctor will also examine you to look for signs of lung cancer and other health problems. If the medical history and physical examination suggest you may have lung cancer, more involved tests will probably be done. These might include imaging tests and/or biopsies of lung tissue.

Imaging Tests

Imaging tests use x-rays, magnetic fields, sound waves, or radioactive substances to create pictures of the inside of your body. Imaging tests may be done for a number of reasons, both before and after a diagnosis of lung cancer:

- to help find a suspicious area that might be cancerous
- to learn how far cancer has spread
- to help determine whether treatment has been effective
- to look for possible signs of cancer recurrence after treatment

Chest x-ray

A chest x-ray is often the first test your doctor will do to look for masses or spots on the lungs. X-rays of your chest can be done at imaging centers, hospitals, and even in some doctors' offices. If the x-ray is normal, you probably do not have lung cancer (although some lung cancers may not show up on an x-ray). If the x-ray reveals any suspicious areas, your doctor may order additional tests.

Computed tomography scan

A **computed tomography** scan (usually called a CT or CAT scan) is a test that uses x-rays to produce detailed cross-sectional images of your body. Instead of taking one picture, as does a conventional x-ray, a CT scanner takes many pictures as it rotates around you. A computer then combines those pictures into an image of a slice of your body. The machine takes pictures and forms multiple images of the part of your body that is being studied. Unlike a regular x-ray, a CT scan creates detailed images of the soft tissues in the body.

Before the CT scan, you may need to drink a **contrast solution** and/or receive an intravenous (IV) injection of a contrast dye that will help outline structures in the body. You may need an IV line for the injection of the contrast dye. The contrast solution may cause some flushing (a feeling of warmth, especially in the face). Some people have an allergic reaction to the dye, which can cause hives or, rarely, more serious reactions, such as trouble breathing or low blood pressure. Be sure to tell the doctor if you have any allergies or you have ever had a reaction to any contrast material used for x-rays.

A CT scan takes longer than a regular x-ray, and it exposes you to a small amount of radiation. You will need to lie still on a table while it is being done. During the test, the table slides in and out of the scanner, a ring-shaped machine that completely surrounds the table. You might feel a bit confined while the pictures are being taken. The test itself is painless, other than any discomfort caused by the insertion of the IV line.

A CT scan can provide precise information about the size, shape, and position of any tumors and can help find enlarged lymph nodes that might contain cancer that has spread from the lung. CT scans are more sensitive than chest x-rays in finding early lung cancers. This test can also be used to look for masses in the adrenal glands, liver, brain, and other internal organs that could be affected by the spread of lung cancer.

CT–guided needle biopsy

If there is a suspicious area deep within the body, a CT scan can be used to guide a biopsy needle precisely into the suspected area. For a **CT–guided needle biopsy**, the person remains on the CT scanning table while the doctor moves a biopsy needle through the skin and toward the location of the mass. CT scans are repeated until the needle is within the mass. A biopsy sample is then removed to be examined under a microscope.

Magnetic resonance imaging

Like CT scans, **magnetic resonance imaging (MRI)** scans provide detailed images of soft tissues in the body. MRIs, however, use radio waves and strong magnets instead of x-rays. The energy from the radio waves is absorbed by the body and then released in a pattern formed by the type of body tissue and by certain diseases. A computer translates the pattern into a detailed image of parts of the body. A contrast material called gadolinium may be injected into a vein before the MRI to better show details.

MRI scans are a little more uncomfortable than CT scans. They take longer—often up to an hour. You will need to lie inside a narrow tube, which is confining and can upset people with a fear of enclosed spaces. Newer, more open MRI machines can help with this concern. The MRI machine makes loud buzzing and clicking noises that you may find disturbing. Some centers provide earplugs to help block out this noise. MRI scans are most often used to look for possible spread of lung cancer to the brain or spinal cord.

Positron emission tomography

For a **positron emission tomography (PET)** scan, a form of radioactive sugar (known as fluorodeoxyglucose or FDG) is injected into the blood. The amount of radioactivity used is very low. Cancer cells in the body absorb the radioactive sugar. After about an hour, you will be moved to a table in the PET scanner. You will need to lie on the table for about 30 minutes while a special camera creates a picture of areas of radioactivity in the body. The picture is not finely detailed like a CT or MRI scan, but it can provide helpful information about your whole body.

The PET scan can be an important test if you appear to have early-stage lung cancer. Your doctor can use this test to determine whether cancer has spread to nearby lymph nodes or other areas, which will affect whether surgery is an option for you. A PET scan can be helpful in determining whether an abnormal area on a chest x-ray is cancer. PET scans are also useful if your doctor thinks the cancer has spread but does not know where. A PET scan can reveal metastasis to the liver, bones, adrenal glands, or some other organs. It is not as useful for looking at the brain, since all brain cells use a lot of glucose.

Some newer machines can perform a PET and CT scan at the same time (PET/CT scan), allowing the doctor to compare areas of higher radioactivity on the PET scan with the more detailed image of that area from the CT scan.

Bone scan

A **bone scan** is used to look for cancer that has spread to the bones. For this test, a small amount of low-level radioactive material is injected into a vein. Over the course of a couple of hours, the substance travels through the bloodstream and settles in areas of bone changes in your skeleton. You then lie on a table for about 30 minutes while a special camera detects the radioactivity and creates a picture of your skeleton. Areas of active bone change attract the radioactivity and show up as "hot spots." These areas may suggest the presence of metastatic cancer, but arthritis or other bone diseases can also cause the same pattern. If an area lights up on the scan, your cancer care team may use other imaging tests, such as simple x-rays or MRIs, to get a better look. If metastatic cancer is suspected, they may take biopsy samples of the bone.

Bone scans are done mainly when there is reason to think the cancer may have spread to the bones (because of symptoms such as bone pain) and other test results are not clear. PET scans can usually show the spread of cancer to bones, so bone scans are not usually needed if a PET scan has been done.

Procedures that Sample Tissues and Cells

Whereas symptoms and results of imaging tests may suggest the presence of lung cancer, a lung cancer diagnosis is made by looking at lung cells under a microscope. The cells can be taken from lung secretions (sputum or phlegm), removed from a suspicious area by a **biopsy** or found in fluid removed from the area around the lung in a procedure called **thoracentesis**. One or more of the tests described in this section may be used to find out whether a mass seen on imaging tests is, indeed, lung cancer. These tests are also used to identify the exact type of lung cancer and to determine how far it has spread.

A pathologist, a doctor who uses laboratory tests to diagnose diseases such as cancer, will examine the cells under a microscope. The results will be described in a pathology report, which is usually available within about a week. If you have any questions about your pathology results or any diagnostic tests, talk to your doctor. You can get a second opinion of your pathology report by having your tissue samples sent to a pathologist at another laboratory recommended by your doctor.

Sputum cytology

In sputum cytology, a sample of sputum (mucus coughed up from the lungs) is examined under a microscope to look for cancer cells. Ideally, early morning samples should be taken 3 days in a row. Sputum cytology is more likely to help find non–small cell lung cancers that start in the major airways of the lung, such as squamous cell lung cancers. It may not be as helpful for finding other types of lung cancer.

Fine needle aspiration biopsy

A needle biopsy can be used to get a sample of cells from a suspicious area (mass). In a **fine needle aspiration (FNA) biopsy**, the skin on the chest where the needle will be inserted is usually numbed with local **anesthesia**. The doctor then guides a thin, hollow needle into the suspicious area while looking at your lungs with either fluoroscopy (which is similar to an x-ray, but the image is shown on a screen instead of on film) or CT scans. Unlike fluoroscopy, CT scans do not give a continuous picture, so the needle is inserted toward the mass, a CT image is taken, and the direction of the needle is guided by that image. This process is repeated a few times until the needle is within the mass.

A small sample of the mass is then sucked into a syringe and sent to a laboratory, where it is examined under the microscope for the presence of cancer cells. In some cases, if the diagnosis is not clear based on the FNA biopsy, a larger needle may be used to remove a slightly bigger piece of lung tissue, a procedure known as a **core needle biopsy**. A needle biopsy may be useful for getting samples from tumors in the outer portions of the lungs, where tests such as bronchoscopy (described on page 46) may not be as helpful.

A possible complication of a needle biopsy is that air can leak out of the lung at the biopsy site and into the space between the lung and the chest wall. This can cause part of the lung to collapse and can cause trouble breathing, a complication called a pneumothorax. A pneumothorax often gets better without any treatment. If not, it is treated by putting a small tube into the chest space and sucking out the air over the course of a day or two, after which it usually heals on its own.

An FNA biopsy may also be done to take samples of lymph nodes around the trachea and bronchi. This procedure can be done during bronchoscopy or endoscopic ultrasound (described on pages 46–47). In this procedure, called a **transtracheal fine needle aspiration** or transbronchial FNA, a thin, hollow needle is inserted through the end of the bronchoscope and through the wall of the trachea or bronchus to sample the nearby lymph nodes.

Bronchoscopy

For this examination, a lighted, flexible fiber-optic tube called a bronchoscope is passed through your mouth or nose and into the trachea and bronchi. The mouth and throat are sprayed first with a numbing medicine. You may also be given medicine through an IV line to make you feel relaxed.

Bronchoscopy can help the doctor find tumors or blockages in the larger airways of the lungs. At the same time, small instruments can be passed down the bronchoscope to take biopsies. The doctor can also take cell samples from the lining of the airways with a small brush (called bronchial brushing) or by rinsing the airways with sterile saltwater (bronchial washing). These tissue and cell samples are then examined under a microscope.

Endobronchial ultrasound

Ultrasound is a type of imaging test that uses sound waves to create pictures of the inside of your body. A small, microphone-like instrument called a transducer emits sound waves and picks up the echoes as they bounce off body tissues. The echoes are converted by a computer into a black and white image on a computer screen.

For an **endobronchial ultrasound**, a bronchoscope is fitted with an ultrasound transducer at its tip and is passed down into the trachea. Prior to the procedure, the patient will be lightly sedated and given local anesthesia. The transducer can be pointed in different directions to examine lymph nodes and other structures in the mediastinum. If the ultrasound reveals suspicious areas, such as enlarged lymph nodes, a hollow needle can be passed through the bronchoscope and guided into these areas to obtain a biopsy. The samples are then sent to a laboratory to be examined under a microscope.

Endoscopic esophageal ultrasound

Endoscopic esophageal ultrasound is similar to endobronchial ultrasound, except the doctor passes an endoscope (a lighted, flexible scope) down the throat and into the esophagus (the tube connecting the throat to the stomach). Prior to the procedure, the patient will be lightly sedated and receive local anesthesia. The esophagus lies just behind the trachea and is close to some lymph nodes inside the chest. Ultrasound images taken from inside the esophagus can be helpful in finding large lymph nodes inside the chest that could contain lung cancer. If enlarged lymph nodes are seen on the ultrasound, a hollow needle can be passed through the endoscope to perform a biopsy. The tissue samples are then sent to a laboratory to be examined under a microscope.

Mediastinoscopy and mediastinotomy

These procedures may be done to examine and take samples from the structures in the mediastinum (the area between the lungs). They are done in an operating room while you are under general anesthesia (in a deep sleep). The main difference between the 2 procedures is in the location and size of the incision.

In **mediastinoscopy,** a small cut is made in the front of the neck and a thin, hollow, lighted tube is inserted into the area behind the sternum (breastbone) and in front of the trachea. Special instruments can be passed through this tube to take tissue samples from the lymph nodes along the trachea and the major bronchial tubes. Examining the samples under a microscope can show whether cancer cells are present.

In **mediastinotomy,** the surgeon makes a slightly larger incision (usually about 2 inches long) next to the breastbone. This approach allows the surgeon to reach lymph nodes that cannot be reached by mediastinoscopy.

Thoracentesis

Thoracentesis is done to find out whether a **pleural effusion**—a buildup of fluid around the lungs—is the result of cancer spreading to the pleura (the lining of the lungs). The buildup might also be caused by other conditions, such as heart failure or an infection.

For this procedure, the skin is numbed and a hollow needle is inserted between the ribs to drain the fluid around the lungs. (In a similar test called pericardiocentesis, fluid is removed from the sac around the heart.) The fluid is checked under a microscope to look for cancer cells. Chemical tests of the fluid are also sometimes useful in distinguishing a **malignant** pleural effusion from a benign one.

If a malignant pleural effusion is diagnosed, thoracentesis may be repeated to remove more fluid. Fluid buildup can keep the lungs from filling with air, so thoracentesis can help the patient breathe better.

Thoracoscopy

Thoracoscopy can be done to find out whether cancer has spread to the space between the lungs and the chest wall or to the linings of these spaces. It can also be used to sample tumors on the outer part of the lung or in nearby lymph nodes and fluid and to assess whether a tumor is growing into nearby tissues or organs. This procedure is not often done to diagnose lung cancer, unless doctors are unable to use procedures such as needle biopsies to get sufficient samples for diagnosis.

Thoracoscopy is done in an operating room while you are under general anesthesia. A small incision is made in the side of the chest wall. Sometimes more than one incision is made. The doctor inserts a lighted tube with a small video camera on the end to view the space between the lungs and chest wall. Using this tool, the doctor can look for cancer deposits on the lining of the lung or chest wall and remove small pieces of tissue to be examined under a microscope. (If certain areas cannot be reached with thoracoscopy, the surgeon may need to make a larger incision in the chest wall, a procedure known as a **thoracotomy**.)

Thoracoscopy can also be used to remove part of a lung as part of treatment for some early-stage lung cancers. This type of operation, known as video-assisted thoracic surgery (VATS), is described in more detail in the "Surgery" section on pages 81–82.

Bone marrow aspiration and biopsy

Bone marrow aspiration and biopsy are not typically done in patients with non–small cell lung cancer. They are used to look for metastasis to the bone marrow (the inner part of the bone where new blood cells are made). These tests may be done for patients thought to have limited stage small cell lung cancer if results of blood tests indicate cancer has spread to bone marrow. The two tests are usually done at the same time.

In **bone marrow aspiration**, you lie on a table (either on your side or on your belly). The skin over the hip is cleaned (samples are most often taken from the hip bone). Then the skin and the surface of the bone are numbed with local **anesthetic**, which may cause a brief stinging or burning sensation. A thin, hollow needle is then inserted into the bone, and a syringe is used to extract a small amount of liquid bone marrow (about 1 teaspoon). Even with anesthesia, most patients still have some brief pain when the marrow is removed.

A **bone marrow biopsy** is usually done just after the aspiration. A small piece of bone and marrow is removed with a slightly larger needle, which is twisted as it is pushed down into the bone. The biopsy will likely cause some brief pain. Once the biopsy is complete, pressure will be applied to the site to stop any bleeding.

Laboratory Tests of Biopsy and Other Samples

Samples collected during biopsies or other tests are sent to a pathology laboratory. There, a doctor examines the samples under a microscope to find out whether they contain cancer and, if so, what type. Special tests may be needed to better classify the cancer. Cancers from other organs can spread to the lungs. It is very important to determine where the cancer started and its exact type. Treatment will differ depending on the type of cancer.

Immunohistochemistry

In immunohistochemistry, very thin slices of the tissue sample are attached to glass microscope slides. The samples are then treated with special **antibodies**, proteins designed to attach only to a substance found in certain cancer cells. If the patient's cancer contains that substance, the antibody will attach to the cells. Chemicals are then added so that antibodies attached to the cells change color. The doctor examining the sample under a microscope can see this color change.

Molecular tests

In some cases, doctors may look for specific gene changes in the cancer cells that might affect how they are best treated. For example, the epidermal growth factor receptor (EGFR) is a protein that sometimes appears in high amounts on the surface of adenocarcinoma cells and helps them grow. Some newer anti-cancer drugs target EGFR, but they seem to work best against lung cancers with certain changes in the EGFR gene. These changes are more common in certain groups, such as non-smokers, women, and Asians. But these drugs do not seem to help people whose cancer cells have changes in the KRAS gene. Many doctors now test for changes in genes such as *EGFR* and *KRAS* to determine whether these newer treatments are likely to be helpful.

About 5% of non–small cell lung cancers have been found to have a rearrangement in a gene called *ALK*. This change is most often seen in nonsmokers (or light smokers) who have the adenocarcinoma subtype of NSCLC. A drug has been developed that targets this gene change, and so now doctors may test some people with adenocarcinoma lung cancers for changes in this gene to see whether this drug may help them.

Newer laboratory tests for other genes or proteins may also help guide the choice of treatment. Some of these tests are described in the section called *"What's New in Lung Cancer Research and Treatment?"*

Blood tests

Blood tests are not used to diagnose lung cancer, but they are done to get a sense of a person's overall health. For example, blood tests are used before surgery to help determine whether a person is healthy enough to have an operation.

A **complete blood count (CBC)** determines whether your blood has normal numbers of various cell types. For example, it can show if you are anemic (have a low number of red blood cells), if you could have trouble with bleeding (because of a low platelet count), or if you are at increased risk for infections (because of a low number of white blood cells). This test will be repeated regularly if you are treated with chemotherapy, because these drugs can affect blood-forming cells of the bone marrow.

Blood tests can help spot abnormalities in some organs, such as the liver or kidneys. For example, if cancer has spread to the liver and bones, it may cause abnormal levels of certain chemicals in the blood, such as abnormally high levels of lactate dehydrogenase (LDH).

Pulmonary function tests

Pulmonary function tests (PFTs) are often done after lung cancer is diagnosed to see how well the lungs are working (for example, to determine whether emphysema or chronic obstructive lung disease is present). These tests are especially important if surgery might be a treatment option. Because surgery to remove part or all of a person's lung results in lower lung capacity, it is important to know how well the person's lungs are working before surgery. Some people with poor lung function (such as those with lung damage from smoking) may not have enough lung reserve to tolerate removing even part of a lung. These tests can help the surgeon decide whether surgery is a good option and, if so, how much of the lung can safely be removed. There are different types of PFTs, but they all basically have the person breathe in and out through a tube that is connected to machines that measure airflow. Sometimes, with non–small cell lung cancer, this test is coupled with a test called an arterial blood gas. In this test, blood is removed from an artery (instead of a vein, as in most blood tests) and tested to determine how much oxygen and carbon dioxide it contains.

How Is Lung Cancer Staged?

Staging is the process of finding out how far a cancer has spread. Your treatment and prognosis depend, to a large extent, on the cancer's stage. The stage of a cancer does not change over time, even if the cancer progresses. A cancer that comes back or spreads is still referred to by the stage it was given at the time it was diagnosed. More information is added to the patient's diagnosis to explain the current disease status as needed. There are actually 2 types of stages:

- The **clinical stage** is based on the results of the physical examination, imaging tests (CT scan, chest x-ray, PET scan, etc.), and tests to sample tissues or cells, which are described in the previous section.

- If you have surgery, your doctor can also determine a **pathologic stage**, which is based on the same factors as the clinical stage, plus what is found in surgery.

The clinical and pathologic stages may be different. For example, during surgery the doctor may find cancer that did not show up on imaging tests, which might give the cancer a more advanced pathologic stage.

Because many patients with lung cancer do not have surgery, the clinical stage is often used when describing the extent of this cancer. However, when it is available, the pathologic stage is likely to be more accurate than the clinical stage, as it uses the additional information obtained at surgery.

Staging of Small Cell Lung Cancer: Limited and Extensive Stage

For small cell lung cancer, most doctors prefer to use a 2-stage system for treatment purposes. The 2-stage system divides small cell lung cancers into **limited stage** and **extensive stage**.

Limited stage usually means that the cancer is only in one side of the chest (called a hemithorax). Limited stage can include one lung and the lymph nodes on the same side of the chest. Lymph nodes above the clavicle (collarbone) are included in limited stage as long as they are on the same side of the chest as the cancer. Some doctors also include lymph nodes at the center of the chest (mediastinal lymph nodes) even when they are closer to the other side of the chest. Most important, the cancer is confined to an area that is small enough to be treated with radiation therapy in one treatment area, or port.

Extensive stage is used to describe cancers that have spread to the other lung, to lymph nodes on the other side of the chest, or to distant organs, including the bone marrow. Many doctors consider small cell lung cancer that has spread to the fluid around the lungs to be extensive stage. About two-thirds of people with small cell lung cancer have extensive disease when their cancer is first found.

Small cell lung cancer is often staged in this way because it helps separate people who may be able to get local treatments such as surgery and/or radiation therapy to try to cure the cancer (limited stage) from those for whom these treatments are not likely to be helpful (extensive stage).

The TNM Staging System

A more formal system to describe the growth and spread of lung cancer is the **American Joint Committee on Cancer (AJCC) TNM staging system**. This system is used more often for non–small cell lung cancer. It is not usually used for small cell lung cancer, mainly because treatment options do not vary much between these detailed stages. The TNM system is based on 3 key pieces of information:

- **T** indicates the size of the main (primary) tumor and whether it has grown into nearby areas.
- **N** describes the spread of cancer to nearby (regional) lymph nodes. Lymph nodes are small bean-shaped collections of immune system cells that help fight infections. Cancer often spreads to the lymph nodes before going to other parts of the body.
- **M** indicates whether the cancer has spread to other organs of the body. The most common sites of metastasis for lung cancer are the brain, bones, adrenal glands, liver, kidneys, and the other lung.

Numbers or letters appear after T, N, and M to provide more details about each of these factors. The numbers 0 through 4 indicate increasing severity.

The letter X means "cannot be assessed because the information is not available."

The TNM staging system is complex and can be difficult for patients (and even some doctors) to understand. If you have any questions about the stage of your cancer, ask your doctor to explain it to you.

T categories for lung cancer

TX: The main (primary) tumor cannot be assessed, or cancer cells were seen on sputum cytology but no tumor can be found.

T0: There is no evidence of a primary tumor.

Tis: The cancer is found only in the top layers of cells lining the air passages. It has not invaded deeper lung tissues. This is also known as **carcinoma in situ**.

T1: The tumor is no larger than 3 cm (slightly less than 1¼ inches), has not reached the membranes that surround the lungs (the visceral pleura), and does not affect the main branches of the bronchi. If the tumor is 2 cm (about ⅘ of an inch) or less across, it is called **T1a**. If the tumor is larger than 2 cm but not larger than 3 cm across, it is called **T1b**.

T2: The tumor has one or more of the following features:

- It is between 3 cm and 7 cm (larger than 3 cm but not larger than 7 cm).

- It involves a main bronchus but is not closer than 2 cm (about ¾ inch) to the carina (the point where the trachea splits into the left and right main bronchi).
- It has grown into the visceral pleura (the membranes that surround the lungs).
- The tumor partially clogs the airways but has not caused the entire lung to collapse or develop pneumonia.

If the tumor is 5 cm or less across, it is called **T2a**. If the tumor is larger than 5 cm (but not larger than 7 cm), it is called **T2b**.

T3: The tumor has one or more of the following features:

- It is larger than 7 cm.
- It has grown into the chest wall, the diaphragm (the breathing muscle that separates the chest from the abdomen), the mediastinal pleura (the membranes surrounding the space between the 2 lungs), or the parietal pericardium (the membranes of the sac surrounding the heart).
- It invades a main bronchus and is closer than 2 cm (about ¾ inch) to the carina, but it does not involve the carina itself.
- It has grown into the airways enough to cause an entire lung to collapse or to cause pneumonia in the entire lung.
- Two or more separate tumor nodules are present in the same lobe of a lung.

T4: The cancer has one or more of the following features:

- A tumor of any size has grown into the mediastinum (the space between the lungs), the heart, the large blood vessels near the heart (such as the aorta), the trachea, the esophagus, the backbone, or the carina.
- Two or more separate tumor nodules are present in different lobes of the same lung.

N categories for lung cancer

NX: Nearby lymph nodes cannot be assessed.

N0: There is no spread to nearby lymph nodes.

N1: The cancer has spread to lymph nodes within the lung and/or around the area where the bronchus enters the lung (the hilar lymph nodes). Affected lymph nodes are on the same side as the primary tumor.

N2: The cancer has spread to lymph nodes around the carina or in the mediastinum. Affected lymph nodes are on the same side as the primary tumor.

N3: The cancer has spread to lymph nodes near the collarbone on either side and/or spread to hilar or mediastinal lymph nodes on the side opposite the primary tumor.

M categories for lung cancer

M0: No spread to distant organs or areas. This includes the other lung, lymph nodes farther away than those mentioned in the N stages on page 59, and other organs or tissues, such as the liver, bones, or brain.

M1a: The tumor has any of the following features:

- The cancer has spread to the other lung.
- Cancer cells are found in the fluid around the lung (a condition called a malignant pleural effusion).
- Cancer cells are found in the fluid around the heart (a condition called a malignant pericardial effusion).

M1b: The cancer has spread to distant lymph nodes or to other organs such as the liver, bones, or brain.

Stage Grouping for Lung Cancer

Once the T, N, and M categories have been assigned, this information is combined to assign an overall stage of 0, I, II, III, or IV. This process is called stage grouping. Some stages are subdivided into A and B. The stages identify cancers that have a similar prognosis and thus are treated in a similar way. Patients with lower stage numbers tend to have a better prognosis.

Occult cancer

TX, N0, M0: Cancer cells are seen in a sample of sputum or other lung fluids, but cancer is not found with other tests, so its location cannot be determined.

Stage 0

Tis, N0, M0: The cancer is found only in the top layers of cells lining the air passages. It has not invaded deeper into other lung tissues and has not spread to lymph nodes or distant sites.

Stage IA

T1a/T1b, N0, M0: The cancer is no larger than 3 cm across, has not reached the membranes that surround the lungs, and does not affect the main branches of the bronchi. It has not spread to lymph nodes or distant sites.

Stage IB

T2a, N0, M0: The cancer has one or more of the following features:

- The main tumor is between 3 cm and 5 cm (larger than 3 cm but not larger than 5 cm).
- The tumor has grown into a main bronchus but is not within 2 cm of the carina (and it is not larger than 5 cm).
- The tumor has grown into the visceral pleura (the membranes surrounding the lungs) and is not larger than 5 cm.
- The tumor is partially clogging the airways (and is not larger than 5 cm).
- The cancer has not spread to lymph nodes or distant sites.

Stage IIA

Three main combinations of categories make up this stage.

T1a/T1b, N1, M0: The cancer is no larger than 3 cm, has not grown into the membranes that surround the lungs, and does not affect the main branches of the bronchi. It has spread to lymph nodes within the lung and/or around the area where the bronchus enters the lung (the hilar lymph nodes). These lymph nodes are on the same side as the cancer. It has not spread to distant sites.

OR

T2a, N1, M0: The cancer has one or more of the following features:

- The main tumor is between 3 cm and 5 cm (larger than 3 cm but not larger than 5 cm).
- The tumor has grown into a main bronchus but is not within 2 cm of the carina (and it is not larger than 5 cm).
- The tumor has grown into the visceral pleura (the membranes surrounding the lungs) and is not larger than 5 cm.
- The tumor is partially clogging the airways (and is not larger than 5 cm).

The cancer has also spread to lymph nodes within the lung and/or around the area where the bronchus enters the lung (the hilar lymph nodes). These lymph nodes are on the same side as the cancer. It has not spread to distant sites.

OR

T2b, N0, M0: The cancer has one or more of the following features:

- The main tumor is between 5 cm and 7 cm (larger than 5 cm but not larger than 7 cm).
- The tumor has grown into a main bronchus but is not within 2 cm of the carina (and it is between 5 cm and 7 cm).
- The tumor has grown into the visceral pleura (the membranes surrounding the lungs) and is between 5 cm and 7 cm.
- The tumor is partially clogging the airways (and is between 5 cm and 7 cm).

The cancer has not spread to lymph nodes or distant sites.

Stage IIB

Two combinations of categories make up this stage.

T2b, N1, M0: The cancer has one or more of the following features:

- The main tumor is between 5 cm and 7 cm (larger than 5 cm but not larger than 7 cm).
- The tumor has grown into a main bronchus but is not within 2 cm of the carina (and it is between 5 cm and 7 cm).

- The tumor has grown into the visceral pleura (the membranes surrounding the lungs) and is between 5 cm and 7 cm.
- The cancer is partially clogging the airways (and is between 5 cm and 7 cm).

It has also spread to lymph nodes within the lung and/or around the area where the bronchus enters the lung (the hilar lymph nodes). These lymph nodes are on the same side as the cancer. It has not spread to distant sites.

OR

T3, N0, M0: The main tumor has one or more of the following features:

- It is larger than 7 cm.
- It has grown into the chest wall, the diaphragm, the mediastinal pleura (the membranes surrounding the space between the lungs), or the parietal pericardium (the membranes of the sac surrounding the heart).
- It invades a main bronchus and is closer than 2 cm (about ¾ inch) to the carina, but it does not involve the carina itself.
- It has grown into the airways enough to cause an entire lung to collapse or to cause pneumonia in the entire lung.
- Two or more separate tumor nodules are present in the same lobe of a lung.

The cancer has not spread to lymph nodes or distant sites.

Stage IIIA

Three main combinations of categories make up this stage.

T1 to T3, N2, M0: The main tumor can be any size. It has **not** grown into the mediastinum, the heart, the large blood vessels near the heart (such as the aorta), the trachea, the esophagus, the backbone, or the carina. It has not spread to different lobes of the same lung. The cancer has spread to lymph nodes around the carina or in the mediastinum. These lymph nodes are on the same side as the main lung tumor. The cancer has not spread to distant sites.

OR

T3, N1, M0: The cancer has one or more of the following features:

- It is larger than 7 cm across.
- It has grown into the chest wall, the diaphragm, the mediastinal pleura (the membranes surrounding the space between the lungs), or the parietal pericardium (the membranes of the sac surrounding the heart).
- It invades a main bronchus and is closer than 2 cm to the carina, but it does not involve the carina itself.
- Two or more separate tumor nodules are present in the same lobe of a lung.
- It has grown into the airways enough to cause an entire lung to collapse or to cause pneumonia in the entire lung.

It has also spread to lymph nodes within the lung and/or around the area where the bronchus enters the lung (the hilar lymph nodes). These lymph nodes are on the same side as the cancer. It has not spread to distant sites.

OR

T4, N0 or N1, M0: The cancer has one or more of the following features:

- A tumor of any size has grown into the mediastinum, the heart, the large blood vessels near the heart (such as the aorta), the trachea, the esophagus, the backbone, or the carina.
- Two or more separate tumor nodules are present in different lobes of the same lung.

It may or may not have spread to lymph nodes within the lung and/or around the area where the bronchus enters the lung (the hilar lymph nodes). Any affected lymph nodes are on the same side as the cancer. It has not spread to distant sites.

Stage IIIB

Two combinations of categories make up this stage.

Any T, N3, M0: The cancer can be of any size. It may or may not have grown into nearby structures or caused pneumonia or lung collapse. It has spread to lymph nodes near the collarbone on either side and/or has spread to hilar or mediastinal lymph nodes on the side opposite the primary tumor. The cancer has not spread to distant sites.

OR

T4, N2, M0: The cancer has one or more of the following features:

- A tumor of any size has grown into the mediastinum, the heart, the large blood vessels near the heart (such as the aorta), the trachea, the esophagus, the backbone, or the carina.
- Two or more separate tumor nodules are present in different lobes of the same lung.

The cancer has also spread to lymph nodes around the carina or in the mediastinum. Affected lymph nodes are on the same side as the main lung tumor. It has not spread to distant sites.

Stage IV

Two combinations of categories make up this stage.

Any T, any N, M1a: The cancer can be any size and may or may not have grown into nearby structures or reached nearby lymph nodes. In addition, any of the following is true:

- The cancer has spread to the other lung.
- Cancer cells are found in the fluid around the lung (called a malignant pleural effusion).

- Cancer cells are found in the fluid around the heart (called a malignant pericardial effusion).

OR

Any T, any N, M1b: The cancer can be any size and may or may not have grown into nearby structures or reached nearby lymph nodes. It has spread to distant lymph nodes or to other organs, such as the liver, bones, or brain.

Lung Cancer Survival Rates by Stage

Survival rates are often used by doctors as a standard way of discussing a person's **prognosis**. Some people may want to know the survival statistics for people in similar situations, while others may not find the numbers helpful or may not want to know them. Whether you want to read about the survival statistics for non–small cell and small cell lung cancer is up to you.

The **5-year survival rate** refers to the percentage of people who live *at least* 5 years after their cancer is diagnosed. Of course, many of these people live much longer than 5 years. To get 5-year survival rates, doctors look at people who were treated at least 5 years ago. Improvements in treatment since then may result in a more favorable outlook for a person now receiving a diagnosis of lung cancer.

Survival rates are often based on previous outcomes of large numbers of people who had the disease, but they cannot predict what will happen to any particular person. Knowing the type and the stage of a person's cancer is important in estimating the person's prognosis. But many other factors may also affect a person's prognosis, such as genetic mutations in the cancer cells, how well the cancer responds to treatment, and a person's overall health. Even when taking these other factors into account, survival rates are at best rough estimates. Your doctor can tell you how these survival rates may apply to you.

Because non–small cell and small cell lung cancer are staged and treated so differently, they have different survival rates. They are presented separately. See page 70 for survival rates for small cell lung cancer.

Survival Rates for Non–Small Cell Lung Cancer

The numbers below are survival rates calculated from the National Cancer Institute's Surveillance, Epidemiology, and End Results (SEER) database, based on people who received a diagnosis of non–small cell lung cancer between 1998 and 2000.

Survival Rates by Stage for Non–Small Cell Lung Cancer

Stage	5-year Survival Rate
IA	49%
IB	45%
IIA	30%
IIB	31%
IIIA	14%
IIIB	5%
IV	1%

Survival Rates for Small Cell Lung Cancer

The numbers below are **relative 5-year survival rates** calculated from the National Cancer Institute's Surveillance, Epidemiology, and End Results (SEER) database, based on people who received a diagnosis of small cell lung cancer between 1988 and 2001. Five-year relative survival rates are adjusted for people who die from causes other than lung cancer. They are considered to be a more accurate way to describe the prognosis for people with a particular type and stage of cancer. These survival rates are based on the TNM staging system in use at the time, which has since been modified slightly. Because of this change, the survival numbers may be slightly different for the latest staging system.

Relative Survival Rates by Stage for Small Cell Lung Cancer

Stage	5-year Relative Survival Rate
I	31%
II	19%
III	8%
IV	2%

Treatment

How Is Lung Cancer Treated?

This section begins with an overview of members of your **cancer care team**. You may see a number of doctors and health care professionals over the course of your diagnosis and treatment, and this section summarizes some of the key professionals who may be part of your care.

Non–small cell lung cancer and small cell lung cancer are treated very differently. If you have received a diagnosis of **non–small cell lung cancer**, go to page 78 to read about treatment options. If you have received a diagnosis of **small cell lung cancer**, go to page 109 to read about treatment options.

Your Cancer Care Team

Your cancer care team comprises several people, each with a different type of expertise to contribute to your care. One of your team members will take the lead in coordinating your care. It should be clear to all team members who is in charge, and that person should inform the others of your progress. This alphabetical list will acquaint you with the health care professionals you may encounter, depending on which treatment option and follow-up path you choose, and their areas of expertise.

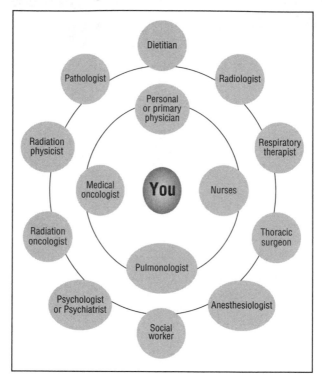

Anesthesiologist

An anesthesiologist is a medical doctor who administers anesthesia (drugs or gases) to render you unconscious or to prevent or relieve pain during and after a surgical procedure.

Dietitian

A dietitian is specially trained to help you make healthy diet choices and maintain a healthy weight before, during, and after treatment. Dietitians can help patients deal with side effects of treatment, such as nausea, vomiting, or sore throat. A registered dietitian (RD) has at least a bachelor's degree and has passed a national competency examination.

Medical oncologist

A medical oncologist (sometimes simply called an oncologist) is a medical doctor you may see after diagnosis. The oncologist is a cancer expert who understands specific types of cancer, their treatments, and their causes. He or she may help cancer patients make decisions about a course of treatment and then manage all phases of cancer care. Oncologists most often become involved when you need chemotherapy, but they can also prescribe hormonal therapy and other anticancer drugs.

Nurses

During your treatment, you will be in contact with different types of nurses.

Case manager: The case manager is usually a nurse or oncology nurse specialist, who coordinates the patient's care throughout diagnosis, treatment, and recovery. The case manager provides guidance through the complex health care system by cutting through red tape, getting responses to questions, managing crises, and connecting the patient and family to needed resources.

Clinical nurse specialist: A clinical nurse specialist (CNS) is a nurse who has a master's degree in a specific area, such as oncology, psychiatry, or critical care nursing. The CNS often provides expertise to staff and may provide special services to patients, such as leading support groups and coordinating cancer care.

Nurse practitioner: A nurse practitioner is a registered nurse with a master's degree or doctoral degree who can manage the care of patients with lung cancer and has additional training in primary care. He or she shares many tasks with your doctors, such as recording your medical history, conducting physical examinations, and doing follow-up care. In most states, a nurse practitioner can prescribe medications with a doctor's supervision.

Oncology-certified nurse: An oncology-certified nurse is a registered nurse who has demonstrated an in-depth knowledge of oncology care. He or she has passed a certification examination. Oncology-certified nurses are found in all areas of cancer practice.

Registered nurse: A registered nurse has an associate's or bachelor's degree in nursing and has passed a state licensing examination. He or she can monitor your condition, provide treatment, educate you about side effects, and help you adjust to cancer, both physically and emotionally.

Pathologist

A pathologist is a medical doctor specially trained in diagnosing disease based on examination of microscopic tissue and fluid samples. He or she will determine the classification (cell type) of your cancer, help determine the stage (extent) and **grade** (estimate of aggressiveness) of your cancer, and issue a pathology report so that you and your doctor can decide on treatment options.

Personal or primary care physician

A personal physician may be a general doctor, internist, or family practice doctor. He or she is often the first medical doctor you saw when you noticed symptoms of illness. This general or family practice doctor may be a member of your medical team, but a specialist is most often a patient's cancer care team leader.

Physician assistant

Physician assistants (PAs) are health care professionals licensed to practice medicine with physician supervision. Physician assistants practice in the areas of primary care medicine (family medicine, internal medicine, pediatrics, and obstetrics and gynecology), as well as in surgery and the surgical subspecialties. Under the supervision of a doctor, they can diagnose and treat medical problems and, in most states, can also prescribe medications.

Psychologist or psychiatrist

A psychologist is a licensed mental health professional who is often part of the cancer care team. He or she provides counseling on emotional and psychological issues. A psychologist may have specialized training and experience in treating people with cancer.

A psychiatrist is a medical doctor specializing in mental health and behavioral disorders. Psychiatrists provide counseling and can also prescribe medications.

Pulmonologist

A pulmonologist is a doctor who specializes in the diagnosis and treatment of lung diseases. A pulmonologist may have first diagnosed your lung cancer, and you may continue to see this doctor if you have breathing trouble related to the cancer or other lung problems.

Radiation oncologist

A radiation oncologist is a medical doctor who specializes in treating cancer by using therapeutic radiation (high-energy x-rays or seeds). If you choose radiation, the radiation oncologist evaluates you frequently during the course of treatment and at intervals afterward. The radiation oncologist will usually work closely with your oncologist and will help you make decisions about radiation therapy options. A radiation oncologist is assisted by a radiation therapist during treatment and works with a radiation physicist, an expert who is trained in ensuring that you receive the correct dose of radiation treatment. The physicist is also assisted by a dosimetrist, a technician who helps plan and calculate the dosage, number, and length of your radiation treatments.

Radiation physicist

A radiation physicist ensures that the radiation machine delivers the right amount of radiation to the correct site in the body. The physicist works with the radiation oncologist to choose the treatment schedule and dose that will have the best chance of killing the most cancer cells.

Radiologist

A radiologist is a medical doctor specializing in the use of imaging procedures (for example, diagnostic x-rays, ultrasound, magnetic resonance images, and bone scans) that produce pictures of internal body structures. He or she has special training in diagnosing cancer and other diseases and interpreting the results of imaging procedures. Your radiologist issues a radiology report describing the findings to your radiation oncologist or oncologist. The radiology images and report may be used to aid in diagnosis; to help classify and determine the extent of your illness; to help locate tumors during procedures, surgery, and radiation treatment; or to look for the possible spread or recurrence of the cancer after treatment.

Respiratory therapist

A respiratory therapist is a health professional who evaluates, treats, or cares for patients with breathing or cardiopulmonary disorders. This person typically works under the direction of a physician to plan and administer respiratory therapy.

Social worker

A social worker is a health specialist, usually with a master's degree, who is licensed or certified by the state in which he or she works. A social worker is an expert in coordinating and providing social services. He or she is trained to help you and your family deal with a range of emotional and practical challenges, such as finances, child care, emotional issues, family concerns and relationships, transportation, and problems with the health care system. If your social worker is trained in cancer-related problems, he or she can counsel you about your fears or concerns, help answer questions about diagnosis and treatment, and lead cancer support groups. You may communicate with your social worker during a hospital stay or on an outpatient basis.

Thoracic surgeon

A thoracic surgeon is a doctor who specializes in performing chest surgery. This doctor will most likely do any tumor biopsies that are part of the lung cancer diagnosis.

How Is Non–Small Cell Lung Cancer Treated?

For treatment information for small cell lung cancer, go to page 109.

General Treatment Information

The next few sections describe the various types of treatments used for non–small cell lung cancer. This information is followed by a description of the most common approaches used for these cancers based on the stage of the cancer.

Making treatment decisions

After the cancer is found and staged, your cancer care team will discuss your treatment options with you. Depending on the stage of the disease and other factors, these are the main treatment options for people with non–small cell lung cancer (NSCLC):

- surgery
- radiation therapy
- other local treatments
- chemotherapy
- targeted therapy

In many cases, more than one of these treatments may be recommended.

It is important to take time and think about your options. In choosing a treatment plan, one of the most important factors is the stage of the cancer. For this reason, it is very important that your doctor order all the tests needed to determine the cancer's stage. Other factors to consider include your overall health, the likely **side effects** of the treatment, and the probability of curing the disease, extending life, or relieving symptoms. Age alone should not be a barrier to treatment. Older people can benefit from treatment as much as younger people, as long as their general health is good.

When considering your treatment options, it is often a good idea to get a second opinion, if possible. A second opinion may provide you with more information and help you feel more confident about the treatment plan you have chosen. Your doctor should not mind that you want to get a second opinion. If your doctor has ordered tests, the results can be sent to the second doctor so that you will not have to have the tests done a second time.

Surgery

Surgery to remove the cancer may be an option for early-stage non–small cell lung cancers, often along with other treatments. If surgery can be done, it provides the best chance to cure NSCLC. Lung cancer surgery is a complex operation that can have serious consequences, so it should be performed by a surgeon who has a lot of experience operating on lung cancers.

If your doctor thinks the lung cancer can be treated with surgery, pulmonary function tests will be done beforehand to determine whether you will have enough healthy lung tissue left after surgery. Other tests will check the function of your heart and other organs to be sure you are healthy enough for surgery.

Types of lung surgery

Several different operations can be used to treat (and possibly cure) non–small cell lung cancer. These operations require general anesthesia (where you are in a deep sleep) and a surgical incision between the ribs in the side of the chest, a procedure called a thoracotomy.

- **pneumonectomy:** surgery in which an entire lung is removed
- **lobectomy:** surgery in which a section (lobe) of the lung is removed
- **segmentectomy or wedge resection:** surgery in which part of a lobe is removed

Another type of operation, known as a **sleeve resection**, may be used to treat some cancers in large airways in the lungs. If you imagine the large airway as the sleeve of a shirt and the tumor as a stain an inch or two above the wrist, a sleeve resection would be like cutting the sleeve above and below the stain and sewing the cuff back onto the shortened sleeve. A surgeon may be able to do this operation instead of a pneumonectomy to preserve more lung function.

With any of these operations, nearby lymph nodes are also removed to look for possible metastasis. The type of operation your doctor recommends will depend on the size and location of the tumor and on your lung function. In some cases, doctors may do a more extensive operation (for example, a lobectomy instead of a segmentectomy) if a person's lungs are healthy enough, as it can provide a better chance to cure the cancer.

When you wake up from surgery, you will have a tube (or tubes) coming out of your chest. These tubes drain fluid and air from around the lungs into a special canister. Some patients will have an air leak after lung surgery. An air leak happens when air from the lung tissue leaks into the chest cavity. Too much air can cause the lung tissue to collapse. Chest tubes prevent this from happening. Air leaks generally resolve within 3 to 5 days of surgery. The tube(s) will be removed once the fluid drainage and air leak subside. Generally, you will need to spend 5 to 7 days in the hospital after the surgery.

Video-assisted thoracic surgery: Some doctors now treat some early-stage lung cancers near the outside of the lung with a procedure called

video-assisted thoracic surgery (VATS), which is less invasive than a thoracotomy. During this operation, a thin, rigid tube with a tiny video camera on the end is inserted through a small hole in the side of the chest, enabling the surgeon to see the chest cavity on a TV monitor. One or two other small incisions are made in the skin, and long instruments are inserted through these holes and used to perform the same operation that would be done in a thoracotomy. If a lobectomy or pneumonectomy is needed, one of the incisions will be enlarged to allow the specimen to be removed. Because only small incisions are typically needed, there is a little less pain after the surgery and a shorter hospital stay—usually 4 to 5 days—than with the more invasive procedures.

Most experts recommend that only early-stage tumors smaller than 3 to 4 centimeters (about 1½ inches) near the outside of the lung be treated this way. The cure rate after this surgery seems to be the same as with older techniques. But it is important that the surgeon performing this procedure is experienced since it requires a great deal of technical skill.

Possible risks and side effects of lung surgery

Possible complications depend on the extent of the surgery and a person's health beforehand. Serious complications can include excessive bleeding, wound infections, and pneumonia. While rare, in some cases, people may not survive the surgery, which is why it is very important that surgeons select patients carefully.

Surgery for lung cancer is a major operation, and recovering from the operation typically takes weeks to months. Because the surgeon must spread ribs to get to the lung when doing a thoracotomy, the incision will hurt for some time after the surgery. Your activity will be limited for at least a month or two.

If your lungs are otherwise in good condition, you can usually return to normal activities after a lobe or even an entire lung has been removed, though it may take some time. If you also have non-cancerous lung diseases, such as emphysema or chronic bronchitis (which are common among heavy smokers), you may become short of breath with activities after surgery.

Surgery for lung cancers with limited spread to other organs

If the lung cancer has spread to the brain or adrenal gland and there is only one metastasis, you may benefit from having the tumor removed. This surgery should be considered only if the tumor in the lung can also be completely removed. Even then, not all lung cancer experts agree with this approach, especially if the tumor is in the adrenal gland.

Tumors in the brain will be removed by craniotomy, surgery through a hole in the skull. It should only be done if the tumor can be removed without damaging vital areas of the brain that control movement, sensation, and speech.

Surgery to relieve symptoms of NSCLC

If you cannot have major surgery because of reduced lung function or other serious medical problems, or if the cancer is too widespread to be cured by surgery, other types of surgery may still be used to relieve some symptoms.

For example, fluid can sometimes build up in the chest cavity outside of the lungs. It can press on the lungs and cause breathing problems. To remove the fluid and keep it from coming back, doctors sometimes perform a procedure called **pleurodesis**. A small cut is made in the skin of the chest wall, and a hollow tube is placed into the chest to remove the fluid. Depending on the situation, talc, a drug such as doxycycline, or a chemotherapy drug is then instilled into the chest cavity. This causes the linings of the lung and chest wall to stick together, sealing the space and limiting further fluid buildup. The tube is generally left in for a couple of days to drain any new fluid that might accumulate.

Other non-surgical techniques can also be used to relieve symptoms. For example, tumors can sometimes grow into airways, blocking them and causing such problems as pneumonia or shortness of breath. Treatments such as **laser therapy** or **photodynamic therapy** can be used to relieve blockages in the airway. In some cases, a bronchoscope may be used to place a stent (a rubber or metal tube) in the airway after treatment to help keep it open. These procedures are described in more detail in the section "Other Local Treatments" on page 90.

Radiation Therapy

Radiation therapy uses high-energy rays (such as x-rays) or particles to kill cancer cells. There are 2 main types of radiation therapy—**external beam radiation therapy** and **brachytherapy (internal radiation** therapy).

External beam radiation therapy

External beam radiation therapy (EBRT) is the most common type of radiation therapy used to treat a primary lung cancer or metastases to other organs. The radiation is delivered from a machine outside the body and focused on the area affected by the cancer.

Before your treatments start, the radiation team will take careful measurements to determine the correct angles for aiming the radiation beams and the proper dose of radiation. Radiation therapy is much like getting an x-ray, but the radiation is stronger. The procedure itself is painless. Each treatment lasts only a few minutes, although the setup time—getting you into place for treatment—usually takes longer. Most often, radiation treatments to the lungs are given 5 days a week for a period of 4 to 7 weeks.

Newer EBRT techniques help doctors treat lung cancers more accurately while reducing radiation exposure to nearby healthy tissues. These techniques may improve the chance of success while reducing side effects. Most doctors now recommend using these newer techniques when they are available.

Three-dimensional conformal radiation therapy (3D-CRT): Three-dimensional conformal radiation therapy (3D-CRT) uses special computers to map precisely the location of the tumor(s). Radiation beams are shaped and aimed at the tumor(s) from several directions, making damage to surrounding healthy tissues less likely.

Intensity-modulated radiation therapy (IMRT): Intensity-modulated radiation therapy (IMRT) is an advanced form of 3D radiation therapy. It uses a computer-driven machine that moves around the patient as it delivers radiation. In addition to shaping the beams and aiming them at the tumor from several angles, this technique allows the intensity of the beams to be adjusted to minimize the amount of radiation that reaches the most sensitive healthy tissues. This technique is often used if tumors are near important structures such as the spinal cord. Many major hospitals and cancer centers are now able to provide IMRT.

Stereotactic radiation therapy: A newer form of treatment, known as stereotactic body radiation therapy (SBRT) or stereotactic ablative radiotherapy (SABR), is sometimes used to treat very early stage lung cancers when surgery is not an option because of issues with the patient's health. Instead of giving small doses of radiation each day for several weeks, SBRT uses focused beams of high-dose radiation given on one or a few days. Several beams are aimed at the tumor from different angles. To target the radiation precisely, the person is put in a specially designed body frame for each treatment. This frame reduces the movement of the lung tumor during breathing. Like other forms of external radiation, the treatment itself is painless. Early results with SBRT have been very promising, and it seems to have a low risk of complications. But because it is still a fairly new technique, there is not much long-term data on its use.

Another type of stereotactic radiation therapy can sometimes be used instead of surgery for single tumors that have spread to the brain. This treatment is sometimes called stereotactic radiosurgery or SRS. In one version of stereotactic body radiation therapy, a machine called a Gamma Knife focuses about 200 beams of radiation on the tumor from different angles over the course of a few minutes to a few hours. The head is placed in a rigid frame to prevent movement. Another type uses a computer-controlled machine called a linear accelerator, which moves around the head to deliver radiation to the tumor from many different angles.

Brachytherapy (internal radiation therapy)

Brachytherapy is used most often to shrink tumors in the airway as a way to relieve symptoms. In some cases, it may be part of a larger treatment regimen aimed at curing the cancer. For this type of treatment, the doctor places a small source of radioactive material (often in the form of a pellet) directly into the cancer or into the airway next to the cancer. This procedure is usually done using a bronchoscope, although it may also be done during surgery. The radiation travels only a short distance from the source, limiting the effects on surrounding healthy tissues. The radiation source is usually removed after a short time. Less often, small radioactive "seeds" are left in place permanently, and the radiation weakens over several weeks.

When is radiation therapy used?

External beam radiation therapy is sometimes used as the main treatment for lung cancer (often with chemotherapy), especially if the person's health is too poor for surgery or the lung tumor cannot be removed by surgery because of its size or location. After surgery, radiation therapy can be used (alone or with chemotherapy) to try to kill very small deposits of cancer that surgery may have missed. In some cases, radiation therapy may be used before surgery (usually with chemotherapy) to try to shrink a lung tumor to make surgery easier.

Radiation therapy can also be used to relieve symptoms of advanced lung cancer, such as pain, bleeding, trouble swallowing, cough, and problems caused by brain metastases. For example, brachytherapy is most often used to help relieve blockages of large airways by cancer.

In some cases, doctors may recommend giving lower doses of radiation to the whole brain, even if there are no visible signs the cancer has spread. This treatment is known as prophylactic cranial irradiation, and its goal is to prevent tumors from forming in the brain. Doctors do not agree, however, that the potential benefits of this treatment outweigh its side effects. If it is used, it is usually given 5 days a week over a 2-week period.

Possible side effects of radiation therapy

Side effects of external radiation therapy can include sunburn-like skin problems and hair loss in the treated area, fatigue, nausea, vomiting, loss of appetite, and weight loss. These side effects often go away after treatment. When radiation is given with chemotherapy, these side effects are often worse.

Radiation therapy to the chest can damage your lungs and cause a cough, breathing problems, and shortness of breath. These symptoms usually improve after treatment is over, although in some cases they may not go away completely. Your esophagus is in the middle of your chest and could be exposed to radiation, which can cause a sore throat and trouble swallowing during treatment. This may make it hard to eat anything other than soft foods or liquids for a while.

Radiation therapy to large areas of the brain can cause memory loss, headaches, trouble thinking, or reduced sexual desire. These symptoms are usually minor in comparison to symptoms caused by a brain tumor, but they can affect your quality of life. Side effects of radiation therapy to the brain usually become most serious 1 or 2 years after treatment.

Other Local Treatments

Treatments other than surgery or radiation therapy may be used to treat lung tumors at certain locations.

Radiofrequency ablation

Radiofrequency ablation (RFA) is being studied for small lung tumors that are near the outer edge of the lungs, especially in people who cannot or do not wish to have surgery. It uses high-energy radio waves to heat the tumor. A thin, needle-like probe is placed through the skin and moved along until the end is in the tumor. Placement of the probe is guided by CT scans. Once the probe is in place, an electric current is passed through it, heating the tumor and destroying the cancer cells. RFA is usually done as an outpatient procedure, using local anesthesia where the probe is inserted. You may also be given medicine to help you relax. Major complications are uncommon, but they can include the partial collapse of a lung (which often resolves on its own) or bleeding into the lung.

Photodynamic therapy

Photodynamic therapy (PDT) is sometimes used to treat very early-stage lung cancers that are still confined to the outer layers of the lung airways or cancers for which other treatments are not appropriate. It can also be used to help open up airways blocked by tumors to help people breathe more easily.

For this technique, a light-activated drug called porfimer sodium (Photofrin) is injected into a vein.

Over the next couple of days, the drug travels throughout the body and collects in cancer cells. A bronchoscope is then passed down the throat and into the lung. This procedure may be done with either local or general anesthesia. A special laser on the end of the bronchoscope is aimed at the tumor and activates the drug, causing the cells to die. The dead cells are removed a few days later during a bronchoscopy. The process can be repeated if needed.

PDT may cause swelling in the airway for a few days, which can lead to some shortness of breath and can cause the person to cough up blood or thick mucus. Some of this drug also collects in normal cells in the body, such as cells in the skin and eyes, which can make you very sensitive to sunlight or strong indoor lights. Too much exposure to light can cause serious skin reactions, so doctors recommend staying out of all strong light for 4 to 6 weeks after the injection.

Laser therapy

Lasers can sometimes be used to treat very small lung cancers in the linings of the airways. They can also be used to help open up airways blocked by larger tumors to help people breathe better. You will usually be under general anesthesia for this type of treatment. The laser is located on the end of a bronchoscope, which is passed down the throat until it is next to the tumor. The doctor then aims the laser beam at the tumor to destroy it. This treatment can usually be repeated, if needed.

Stent placement

Lung tumors that have grown into an airway can cause trouble breathing or other problems. To help keep the airway open, doctors may place a stent in the airway. This procedure may be done after such treatments as photodynamic therapy or laser therapy. Stents are hard silicone or metal tubes that can be put in place in the airway with a bronchoscope.

Chemotherapy

Chemotherapy is treatment with cancer-killing drugs that are given intravenously (injected into a vein) or by mouth. It is a type of systemic therapy, meaning the drugs travel through the bloodstream to reach cancer cells throughout the body, making this treatment useful for cancer that has metastasized to distant organs. Depending on the stage of lung cancer, chemotherapy may be used in different situations:

- to try to shrink a tumor before surgery, sometimes with radiation therapy. This use is known as **neoadjuvant therapy**.
- after surgery, to try to kill cancer cells that may have been left behind. This use is known as **adjuvant therapy**.
- as the main treatment (sometimes with radiation therapy) for advanced cancers or for people who cannot withstand surgery.

Doctors give chemotherapy in cycles, with each treatment period (usually 1 to 3 days) followed by a rest period to allow the body time to recover. Some chemotherapy drugs, however, may be given every day. Chemotherapy cycles generally last about 3 to 4 weeks, and treatment typically involves 4 to 6 cycles. Chemotherapy may not be recommended for people in poor health, but advanced age by itself is not a barrier to receiving chemotherapy.

Treatment for lung cancer usually uses a combination of 2 chemotherapy drugs. Studies have shown that adding a third chemotherapy drug does not add much benefit and is likely to cause more side effects. Single-drug chemotherapy is sometimes used for people who might not tolerate combination chemotherapy well, such as people whose overall health is poor.

These are the chemotherapy drugs most frequently used for non–small cell lung cancer:

- cisplatin
- carboplatin
- paclitaxel
- docetaxel
- gemcitabine
- vinorelbine
- irinotecan
- etoposide
- vinblastine
- pemetrexed

In the most common combinations, patients receive either cisplatin or carboplatin plus one other drug. Sometimes, combinations with less severe side effects, such as gemcitabine with vinorelbine or paclitaxel, may be used. For people with advanced lung cancer who meet certain criteria, targeted therapy drugs such as bevacizumab (Avastin) or cetuximab (Erbitux) may be added to initial treatment (see the "Targeted Therapies" section on page 96).

If the initial chemotherapy treatment for advanced lung cancer is no longer working, the doctor may recommend second-line treatment with a single drug such as docetaxel or pemetrexed. Another option may be the targeted therapy erlotinib (Tarceva). Advanced age is not a barrier to receiving these drugs as long as the person is in good general health.

Some doctors may recommend second-line treatment with a single chemotherapy or targeted therapy even in people who have responded well to their initial chemotherapy. The intent is to delay growth or recurrence for as long as possible and, hopefully, to help patients live longer. This concept, known as maintenance therapy, is still being studied, as it is not yet clear whether possible benefits outweigh the risks and side effects. For more information, see the chapter "Latest Research," beginning on page 153.

Possible side effects of chemotherapy

Chemotherapy drugs work by attacking cells that are dividing quickly, which is why they work against cancer cells. But other cells in the body, such as those in the bone marrow (where new blood cells are made), the lining of the mouth and intestines, and the hair follicles, also divide quickly. These cells are also likely to be affected by chemotherapy, which can lead to side effects.

The side effects of chemotherapy depend on the type and dose of drugs given and the length of time they are taken. These are some possible side effects of chemotherapy:

- hair loss
- mouth sores
- loss of appetite
- nausea and vomiting
- diarrhea or constipation
- increased chance of infection (because of low white blood cell counts)
- easy bruising or bleeding (because of low blood platelet counts)
- fatigue (because of low red blood cell counts)

These side effects are usually short-term and go away after treatment is finished. There are often ways to lessen these side effects. For example, there are drugs that can help prevent or reduce nausea and vomiting.

Some drugs, such as cisplatin, vinorelbine, docetaxel, or paclitaxel, can damage nerves. This nerve damage can lead to symptoms, particularly in the hands and feet, such as pain, burning or tingling sensations, sensitivity to cold or heat, and weakness. This is called peripheral neuropathy. In most cases, peripheral neuropathy goes away once treatment is stopped, but it may be longer lasting in some people. For more information, contact the American Cancer Society at **800-227-2345** and request the document *Peripheral Neuropathy*

Caused by Chemotherapy or visit the Web site, **cancer.org**.

You should report peripheral neuropathy or any other side effects you notice while you are undergoing chemotherapy to your cancer care team so that the side effects can be promptly treated. In some cases, the doses of the chemotherapy drugs may need to be reduced or treatment may need to be delayed or stopped to prevent side effects from getting worse.

For more information about chemotherapy, call **800-227-2345** and request the document *Understanding Chemotherapy: A Guide for Patients and Families* or visit the Web site, **cancer.org**.

Targeted Therapies

As researchers have learned more about the changes in lung cancer cells that help them grow, they have been able to develop newer drugs that specifically target these changes. These **targeted therapies** work differently from standard chemotherapy drugs. Targeted therapies often have different and less severe side effects. Currently, they are used most often for advanced lung cancer, either with chemotherapy or alone.

Drugs that target tumor blood vessel growth

For tumors to grow, they must form new blood vessels to keep them nourished. This process is called **angiogenesis**. Some targeted drugs block this new blood vessel growth.

Bevacizumab (Avastin): Bevacizumab is a type of drug known as a **monoclonal antibody**

(a man-made version of a specific immune system protein). It targets vascular endothelial growth factor (VEGF), a protein that helps new blood vessels form. Bevacizumab has been shown to prolong survival of patients with advanced lung cancer when it is added to standard chemotherapy regimens as part of first-line treatment. Bevacizumab is given by IV infusion every 2 to 3 weeks. Chemotherapy plus bevacizumab is usually given for 4 to 6 cycles. Many doctors, however, continue giving bevacizumab by itself until the cancer starts growing again.

Bevacizumab's possible side effects are different from (and may add to) those caused by chemotherapy drugs. Some of these effects can be serious. Bevacizumab can cause serious bleeding, which limits its use to some extent. It is typically not used in patients who are coughing up blood or who are on blood thinners, such as aspirin or warfarin (Coumadin). Most current guidelines do not recommend bevacizumab for people who have squamous cell lung cancer, because it can lead to serious bleeding in the lungs. Studies are under way to determine whether bevacizumab is safe in cases in which the cancer is not located near large blood vessels in the center of the chest.

Other rare but possibly serious side effects include blood clots, holes forming in the intestines, heart problems, and slow wound healing. More common side effects include high blood pressure, tiredness, low white blood cell counts, headaches, mouth sores, loss of appetite, and diarrhea.

Drugs that target epidermal growth factor receptor

Epidermal growth factor receptor (EGFR) is a protein found on the surface of cells. It normally helps the cells to grow and divide. Some lung cancer cells have too much EGFR, which causes them to grow faster.

Erlotinib (Tarceva): Erlotinib is a drug that blocks EGFR from signaling the cells to grow. It has been shown to help keep some lung tumors under control, especially in women and in people who have never smoked. It is used by itself, mainly for people with advanced lung cancer in which initial treatment with chemotherapy is no longer working. Erlotinib may also be used as the first treatment in people whose cancers have a mutation in the *EGFR* gene.

This drug is taken daily as a pill. The side effects of erlotinib tend to be milder than those of typical chemotherapy drugs. The most worrisome side effect for many people is an acne-like rash on the face and chest, which in some cases can lead to skin infections. Other side effects can include diarrhea, loss of appetite, and tiredness.

Cetuximab (Erbitux): Cetuximab is a monoclonal antibody that targets EGFR. For people with advanced lung cancer, some doctors may add it to standard chemotherapy as part of first-line treatment. Cetuximab is not currently approved by the **U.S. Food and Drug Administration (FDA)** for use against lung cancer. It is approved, however, for use against other types of cancer, and doctors can prescribe it to treat lung cancer. This drug is expensive, and not all insurance companies cover the cost. If you are considering taking this drug, it is important to find out beforehand whether your insurance will cover it.

Cetuximab is given by IV infusion, usually once a week. A rare but serious side effect of cetuximab is an allergic reaction during the first infusion, which could cause breathing problems and low blood pressure. You may be given medicine before treatment to help prevent this reaction. Many people develop an acne-like rash on the face and chest during treatment, which in some cases can lead to infections. Other possible side effects include headaches, tiredness, fever, and diarrhea.

For more detailed information on the skin problems that can result from anti-EGFR drugs, contact the American Cancer Society at **800-227-2345** and request the document *Targeted Therapy*, or visit the Web site, **cancer.org**.

Drugs that target the ALK gene

About 5% of non–small cell lung cancers have been found to have a rearrangement in a gene called *ALK*. This change is most often seen in nonsmokers (or light smokers) who have the adenocarcinoma subtype of NSCLC. The *ALK* gene rearrangement produces an abnormal protein that causes the cells to grow and spread. The new drug crizotinib (Xalkori) blocks the abnormal ALK protein. In studies of people whose lung cancers had this gene change, this drug shrank tumors in about

50% to 60% of patients, even though most of them had already had chemotherapy.

The most common side effects are mild and include nausea and vomiting, diarrhea, constipation, swelling, fatigue, and eye problems. Some side effects can be severe, such as low white blood cell counts, lung inflammation, and heart rhythm problems. In August 2011, crizotinib was approved by the FDA to treat patients with lung cancers that have the *ALK* gene change. It is taken twice a day as a pill. While this drug helps shrink tumors, it still is not known whether it helps people live longer. More studies are needed.

Treatment Choices by Stage for Non–Small Cell Lung Cancer

The treatment options for non–small cell lung cancer (NSCLC) are based mainly on the stage of the cancer, but factors such as a person's overall health and lung function and certain traits of the cancer itself are also important.

If you smoke, one of the most important things you can do to be ready for treatment is to try to quit. Studies have shown that people who stop smoking after a lung cancer diagnosis tend to have better outcomes than those who continue to smoke.

Occult cancer

For occult cancers, malignant cells can be seen on sputum cytology but no obvious tumor can be found with bronchoscopy or imaging tests. These cancers are usually early-stage cancers. Bronchoscopy is usually repeated about every 3 months to look for a tumor. If a tumor is found, treatment will depend on the stage.

Stage 0

Because stage 0 NSCLC is limited to the lining of the airways and has not grown deeper into the lung tissue or other areas, it is usually curable by surgery alone. No chemotherapy or radiation therapy is needed.

If you are healthy enough for surgery, you can usually be treated by segmentectomy or wedge resection (removal of defined segments or small wedges of the lung). Cancers in some locations, such as where the trachea divides into the left and right main bronchi, may be treated with a sleeve resection, but these tumors may be hard to remove completely without removing a lobe or the entire lung.

In some cases, photodynamic therapy, laser therapy, or brachytherapy may be useful alternatives to surgery for stage 0 cancers. If your cancer is truly stage 0, these treatments will probably cure you.

Stage I

If you have stage I NSCLC, surgery may be the only treatment you need. The tumor may be removed either by lobectomy or by a procedure that takes out a smaller piece of lung, such as sleeve resection, segmentectomy, or wedge resection. Some lymph nodes within the lung and outside the lung in the mediastinum will be removed to check for cancer cells.

Segmentectomy or wedge resection is recommended only for treating the smallest of stage I cancers (those less than 2 cm across) and for patients with medical conditions that make removing the entire lobe dangerous. These smallest of stage I cancers are most likely to be candidates for video-assisted thoracic surgery (VATS). Most surgeons believe it is better to perform a lobectomy if the patient can tolerate it, as it offers the best chance for cure.

For some people with stage I NSCLC, adjuvant chemotherapy may lower the risk of recurrence, but doctors are not sure how best to determine in which people the benefits outweigh the downsides. Therefore, most do not recommend chemotherapy if it looks like all of the cancer was removed with surgery. New laboratory tests that look at the patterns of certain genes in cancer cells appear promising and may help doctors identify the best candidates for adjuvant chemotherapy in the future. Studies are now under way to determine whether these tests are accurate.

After surgery, if the pathology report reveals there were cancer cells at the edge of the surgical specimen (meaning some cancer could have been left behind), chemotherapy and/or radiation therapy may be recommended. Another approach would be to have a second surgery to ensure that the cancer has been completely removed. (This procedure might also be followed by chemotherapy.)

If you have serious medical problems that would prevent you from having surgery, you may receive only radiation therapy as your main treatment. Radiofrequency ablation (RFA) may be an option if the tumor is small and in the outer part of the lung.

Stage II

People who have stage II NSCLC and are healthy enough for surgery usually have the cancer removed by lobectomy, sleeve resection, or, less frequently, segmentectomy. Sometimes pneumonectomy (removing the whole lung) is needed. Any lymph nodes likely to contain cancer are also removed. The extent of lymph node involvement and whether cancer cells are found at the edges of the removed tissues are important in planning the next step of treatment. In some cases, neoadjuvant chemotherapy (often with radiation) may be recommended to try to shrink the tumor before surgery.

After surgery, chemotherapy (sometimes with radiation therapy) is typically recommended to try to destroy any remaining cancer cells. As with stage I cancers, newer laboratory tests now being studied may allow doctors to determine which patients would benefit most from this adjuvant treatment.

If cancer cells are found at the edge of the tissue removed by surgery, chemotherapy and radiation therapy are more likely to be used. Alternatively, your doctor may recommend a second, more extensive surgery, followed by chemotherapy.

If you have serious medical problems that would prevent you from having surgery, you may receive radiation therapy alone as your main treatment.

Stage IIIA

Treatment for stage IIIA NSCLC may include radiation therapy, chemotherapy, surgery, or some combination of the three. Planning treatment for stage IIIA NSCLC will often require input from a medical oncologist, radiation oncologist, and thoracic surgeon. Treatment options will depend on the size of the tumor, its location, which lymph nodes it has spread to, your overall health, and how well you can tolerate treatment.

For patients who can tolerate it, treatment usually starts with chemotherapy, with or without radiation therapy. Surgery may be an option afterward if the doctor thinks any remaining cancer can be removed and the person is healthy enough. (In selected stage IIIA cancers in which the cancer has not reached the lymph nodes in the mediastinum, surgery may be an option as the first treatment.) Surgery is often followed by chemotherapy, and possibly radiation therapy if it has not been given beforehand.

For people with stage IIIA NSCLC who cannot tolerate chemotherapy or surgery, radiation therapy is usually the treatment of choice.

Stage IIIB

Stage IIIB NSCLC has usually spread too widely to be removed completely by surgery. Treatment will depend on a person's overall health and how well he or she can tolerate treatment. If you are in fairly good health, you may be helped by chemotherapy and radiation therapy. For people who cannot have chemotherapy, radiation therapy is usually the treatment of choice.

Because treatment is unlikely to cure stage IIIB cancers, taking part in a clinical trial of newer treatments could be a good option. Several clinical trials are in progress to determine the best treatment for people with this stage of lung cancer.

Stage IV

Stage IV NSCLC is widespread when it is diagnosed. Because these cancers have spread to distant sites, they are very hard to cure. Treatment options depend on the sites of metastasis, the number of tumors, and your overall health. If you are in otherwise good health, treatments such as surgery, chemotherapy, and radiation therapy may help you live longer and relieve symptoms, even though they are not likely to cure your cancer. Other treatments, such as photodynamic therapy or laser therapy, may also be used to help relieve symptoms. Before starting treatment for advanced NSCLC, be sure you understand the goals of that treatment plan.

Cancer that has spread widely throughout the body is usually treated with chemotherapy, as long as the person is healthy enough to tolerate it. The targeted therapy bevacizumab (Avastin) is FDA-approved for use with chemotherapy in people who are not at high risk for bleeding— for example, those who do not have squamous cell NSCLC, have not coughed up blood, and are not taking blood thinners. Some doctors may use bevacizumab for certain patients with squamous cell cancer if the tumor is not near large blood vessels in the center of the chest. If bevacizumab is used, it is often continued even after chemotherapy is finished.

Other targeted drugs may also be useful in some situations. For tumors that have the *ALK* gene change, crizotinib (Xalkori) is an option. For some others, adding the anti-EGFR drug cetuximab (Erbitux) to chemotherapy may be an option, especially in people who cannot take bevacizumab. For people whose cancers have certain mutations in the *EGFR* gene, some doctors may recommend using the anti-EGFR drug erlotinib (Tarceva) by itself as the first treatment. In some people with those gene changes, chemotherapy may be given first, followed by erlotinib. This approach is known as maintenance therapy.

For cancers that have caused a malignant pleural effusion (fluid in the space around the lungs), the fluid may be drained and pleurodesis may be done to help prevent it from building back up. Then chemotherapy and/or targeted drugs may be given.

Cancer that is not very widespread in the lungs and has only spread to one other site (such as the brain) is not common but can sometimes be treated with surgery and/or radiation therapy. For example, a single tumor in the brain may be treated with surgery or stereotactic radiation (such as the

Gamma Knife), followed by radiation to the whole brain. Treatment for the lung tumor is then based on its T and N stages and may include surgery and/or chemotherapy.

As with other stages, treatment for stage IV non–small cell lung cancer depends on a person's overall health and how well he or she tolerates treatment. For example, some people not in good health might get only 1 chemotherapy drug instead of 2. For people who cannot tolerate chemotherapy, radiation therapy is usually the treatment of choice. Local treatments such as laser therapy, photodynamic therapy, or stent placement may also be used to help relieve symptoms caused by lung tumors.

Because treatment is unlikely to cure these cancers, taking part in a clinical trial of newer treatments may be a good option.

Cancer that progresses or recurs after treatment

If cancer continues to grow during treatment or comes back, further treatment will depend on the extent of the cancer, what treatments have been used, and the person's health and desire for further treatment. It is important to understand the goal of any further treatment—whether to try to cure the cancer, slow its growth, or help relieve symptoms—as well as the likelihood of benefits and risks.

If cancer continues to grow during initial treatment with radiation therapy, chemotherapy may be tried. If a cancer continues to grow during combination chemotherapy, second line treatment most often consists of a single chemotherapy drug, such as docetaxel or pemetrexed, or the targeted therapy erlotinib (Tarceva).

Smaller cancers that recur locally in the lungs can sometimes be retreated with surgery or radiation therapy (if it has not already been used). Cancers that recur in the lymph nodes between the lungs are usually treated with chemotherapy, possibly along with radiation (if it has not already been used). For cancers that return at distant sites, chemotherapy and/or targeted therapies are often the treatments of choice.

At some point, it may become clear that standard treatments are no longer controlling the cancer. If you want to continue anti-cancer treatment, you might think about taking part in a clinical trial of newer lung cancer treatments. While clinical trials are not always the best option for every person, they may benefit you, as well as future patients.

Even if your cancer cannot be cured, treatment can help you be as free of symptoms as possible. If curative treatment is not an option, treatment aimed at specific sites can often relieve symptoms and may even slow the spread of the disease. Symptoms that are caused by cancer in the airways—such as shortness of breath or coughing up blood—can often be treated effectively with radiation therapy, brachytherapy, laser therapy, photodynamic therapy, stent placement, or even surgery. Radiation therapy can be used to help control metastasis in the brain or relieve pain in a specific area if the cancer has spread.

Many people with lung cancer are concerned about pain. Cancer growing near certain nerves can sometimes cause pain, but this can almost always be treated effectively with pain medicines. Sometimes radiation therapy or other treatments can help control pain. It is important that you talk to your doctor and take advantage of treatments that could improve your quality of life.

It is never easy to decide on the right time to stop treatment aimed at curing the cancer and start focusing on care that relieves symptoms. Good communication with doctors, nurses, family, friends, and clergy can often help people facing this situation.

For information on clinical trials and complementary and alternative treatments, see pages 126 and 134.

How Is Small Cell Lung Cancer Treated?

For treatment information for non–small cell lung cancer, go to page 78.

General Treatment Information

The next few sections describe the various types of treatments used for small cell lung cancer. This information is followed by a description of the most common approaches used for these cancers based on the stage of the cancer.

Making treatment decisions

Depending on the stage of the disease and other factors, these are the main treatment options for people with small cell lung cancer (SCLC):

- surgery
- radiation therapy
- chemotherapy

If you have small cell lung cancer and you are healthy enough to tolerate it, you will probably undergo chemotherapy. If you have limited stage disease, radiation therapy and—rarely—surgery may be options as well.

After the cancer is found and staged, your cancer care team will discuss your treatment options with you. It is important to take time to think about your choices. The stage of the cancer is one of the most important factors to consider when choosing a treatment plan. For this reason, it is very important that your doctor order all the tests needed to determine the cancer's stage. Other factors to consider include your overall health, the likely side effects of treatment, and the probability of curing the disease, extending life, or relieving symptoms. Age alone should not be a barrier to treatment. Older people can benefit from treatment just as much as younger people as long as their general health is good.

Surgery

Surgery is rarely used as the main form of treatment in small cell lung cancer. Occasionally (in fewer than 1 of 20 cases), the cancer is found as only one localized tumor nodule with no spread to lymph nodes or other organs. Surgery may be an option in these cases, usually followed by additional treatment (chemotherapy, often with radiation therapy).

If your doctor thinks your lung cancer can be treated with surgery, pulmonary function tests will be done beforehand to determine whether you will have enough healthy lung tissue left after surgery. Other tests will check the function of your heart and other organs to be sure you are healthy enough for surgery.

Because more advanced lung cancers will not be helped by surgery, your doctor will also want to make sure the cancer has not spread to the lymph nodes between the lungs. This assessment can be done before surgery with mediastinoscopy or with some of the other techniques described in the section "How Is Lung Cancer Diagnosed?" beginning on page 33.

Types of lung surgery

Several different operations can be used to treat small cell lung cancer. These operations require general anesthesia (in which you are in a deep sleep) and a surgical incision between the ribs in the side of the chest, a procedure called a thoracotomy.

- **Pneumonectomy:** surgery in which an entire lung is removed
- **Lobectomy:** surgery in which a section (lobe) of the lung is removed

- **Segmentectomy or wedge resection:**
  surgery in which part of a lobe is removed
- **Sleeve resection:** surgery in which a
  section of a large airway is removed and the
  lung is reattached

In general, lobectomy is the preferred surgery for small cell lung cancers. With any of these operations, nearby lymph nodes are also removed to look for possible metastasis. You will generally need to spend about a week in the hospital after a lobectomy.

Video-assisted thoracic surgery

Some doctors now treat some early-stage small cell lung cancers near the outside of the lung with a procedure called video-assisted thoracic surgery (VATS), which is less invasive than a thoracotomy. During this procedure, a thin, hollow tube with a tiny video camera on the end is inserted through a small hole in the side of the chest, enabling the surgeon to see the chest cavity on a TV monitor. One or two other small incisions are made in the skin, and long instruments are inserted though these holes and used to cut away the tumor. If a lobectomy or pneumonectomy is needed, one of the incisions will be enlarged to remove the lung specimen. Because only small incisions are typically needed, there is a little less pain after surgery and a shorter hospital stay, usually around 4 to 5 days.

Most experts recommend that only tumors smaller than 3 to 4 centimeters (about 1½ inches) near the outside of the lung be removed this way.

The cure rate after this surgery seems to be the same as with older techniques. It is important, however, that the surgeon be experienced with this procedure since it requires a great deal of technical skill.

Possible risks and side effects of lung surgery

Possible complications depend on the extent of the surgery and a person's health beforehand. Serious complications can include excessive bleeding, wound infections, and pneumonia. While rare, in some cases, people may not survive the surgery, which is why it is very important that surgeons select patients carefully.

Surgery for lung cancer is a major operation, and recovery typically takes weeks to months. Because the surgeon must spread the ribs to get to the lung when doing a thoracotomy, the incision will hurt for some time after surgery. Your activity will be limited for at least a month.

If your lungs are otherwise in good condition, you can usually return to normal activities after a lobe or even an entire lung has been removed, though it may take some time. If you also have non-cancerous lung diseases, such as emphysema or chronic bronchitis (which are common among heavy smokers), you may become short of breath with activities after surgery.

Surgery and other techniques to relieve symptoms of SCLC

In some cases, surgery or other localized techniques may be used to help treat the symptoms of the cancer (as opposed to trying to remove all of the cancer). For example, tumors can sometimes grow into and block airways, causing such problems as pneumonia or shortness of breath. Treatments such as laser surgery can be used to relieve blockages in the airway. With laser surgery, a bronchoscope with a special type of laser is used to destroy the cancer cells. In some cases, a bronchoscope may also be used to place a stent (a metal or silicone tube) in the airway after treatment to help keep it open. Other techniques, such as radiation therapy (described on page 85), may also be used.

Sometimes fluid can build up in the chest cavity outside of the lungs. This fluid can press on the lungs and cause breathing problems. To remove the fluid and prevent it from building back up, doctors sometimes perform a procedure called pleurodesis. A small cut is made in the skin of chest wall, and a hollow tube is placed into the chest to remove the fluid. Talc or a drug such as doxycycline or a chemotherapy drug is then instilled into the chest cavity. This causes the linings of the lung (the visceral pleura) and chest wall (the parietal pleural) to stick together, sealing the space and limiting further fluid buildup. The tube is generally left in place for a couple of days to drain any new fluid that might accumulate.

Radiation Therapy

Radiation therapy uses high-energy rays (such as x-rays) or particles to kill cancer cells. The type of radiation therapy most often used to treat small cell lung cancer is external beam radiation therapy. In external beam radiation therapy (EBRT), radiation is delivered from a machine outside the body and focused on the area affected by the cancer.

In SCLC, radiation therapy may be used in several situations. It is most often given with chemotherapy for patients with limited stage disease to treat the tumor and lymph nodes in the chest. After chemotherapy, radiation therapy is sometimes used to kill any small deposits of cancer that may remain. Radiation therapy can also be used to shrink tumors as a means to relieve such symptoms as bone pain, bleeding, trouble swallowing, cough, shortness of breath, and problems caused by brain metastases. In limited stage SCLC, radiation therapy is often given to the brain after other treatments to help reduce the likelihood of metastasis to the brain. This procedure is called prophylactic cranial irradiation.

Before your treatments begin, the radiation team will take careful measurements to find the correct angles for aiming the radiation beams and the proper dose of radiation. Radiation therapy is much like getting an x-ray, but the radiation is stronger. The procedure itself is painless. Each treatment lasts only a few minutes, although the setup time—getting you into place for treatment—usually takes longer. Most often, radiation treatments as part of the initial treatment for SCLC are given once or twice daily, 5 days a week, for 3 to 7 weeks. Radiation to relieve symptoms and prophylactic cranial irradiation are given for shorter periods of time.

Newer EBRT techniques help doctors treat lung cancers more accurately while lowering the radiation exposure to nearby healthy tissues. These techniques may improve the chances of successful treatment while reducing side effects. Most doctors now recommend using these newer techniques when they are available.

Three-dimensional conformal radiation therapy

Three-dimensional conformal radiation therapy (3D-CRT) uses special computer programs to precisely map the location of the tumor(s). Radiation beams are shaped and aimed at the tumor(s) from several directions, making damage to surrounding healthy tissues less likely.

Intensity-modulated radiation therapy

Intensity-modulated radiation therapy (IMRT) is an advanced form of 3D radiation therapy. It uses a computer-driven machine that moves around the patient as it delivers radiation. In addition to shaping the beams and aiming them at the tumor(s) from several angles, this technique allows the intensity of the beams to be adjusted to minimize the amount of radiation that reaches the surrounding healthy tissues. This technique is often used if tumors are near important structures such as the spinal cord. Many major hospitals and cancer centers are now able to provide IMRT.

Possible side effects of radiation therapy

Side effects of radiation therapy can include sunburn-like skin problems and hair loss in the treated area, fatigue, nausea, vomiting, loss of appetite, and weight loss. These side effects often go away after treatment. Radiation can also make the side effects of chemotherapy worse.

Radiation therapy to the chest can damage your lungs, causing a cough, breathing problems, and shortness of breath. These symptoms usually improve after treatment is over, although in some cases they may not go away completely. Your esophagus is in the middle of your chest and could be exposed to radiation, which can cause a sore throat and trouble swallowing during treatment. This may make it hard to eat anything other than soft foods or liquids for a while.

Radiation therapy to large areas of the brain can cause memory loss, headaches, difficulty thinking, or reduced sexual desire. These symptoms are usually minor in comparison to symptoms caused by a brain tumor, but they can affect your quality of life. Side effects of radiation therapy to the brain usually become most serious 1 to 2 years after treatment. Most side effects improve and go away after treatment is completed, but some can be long-lasting or even permanent.

For more information about radiation therapy, visit our Web site at **cancer.org** or call **800-227-2345** and request the document *Understanding Radiation Therapy: A Guide for Patients and Families.*

Chemotherapy

Chemotherapy is treatment with cancer-killing drugs that are given intravenously (injected into a vein) or taken by mouth. It is a type of systemic therapy, meaning the drugs enter the bloodstream and travel throughout the body, making this treatment useful for cancer that has metastasized to organs beyond the lungs. Chemotherapy is usually the main treatment for small cell lung cancer (SCLC).

Doctors give chemotherapy in cycles, with a period of treatment (usually 1 to 3 days) followed by a rest period to allow the body time to recover. Chemotherapy cycles generally last about 3 to 4 weeks, and initial treatment typically is 4 to 6 cycles. Chemotherapy may not be recommended for people in poor health, but advanced age by itself is not a barrier to receiving chemotherapy.

Chemotherapy for SCLC generally uses a combination of 2 drugs. These are the drug combinations most often used for initial chemotherapy for SCLC:

- cisplatin and etoposide
- carboplatin and etoposide
- cisplatin and irinotecan
- carboplatin and irinotecan
- cyclophosphamide, doxorubicin (Adriamycin), and vincristine

If the cancer progresses during treatment or returns after treatment, different chemotherapy drugs may be tried. The choice of drugs depends to some extent on how soon the cancer begins to grow again. The longer it takes for the cancer to return, the more likely it is to respond to further treatment.

- If the cancer progresses during treatment or relapses within 2 to 3 months of finishing treatment, drugs such as topotecan, ifosfamide, paclitaxel, docetaxel, irinotecan, or gemcitabine may be tried.
- If the relapse occurs from 2 to 3 months to 6 months after treatment, topotecan is often the drug of choice. Other drugs that may be tried include irinotecan, the CAV regimen (cyclophosphamide, doxorubicin, and vincristine), gemcitabine, paclitaxel, docetaxel, oral etoposide, or vinorelbine.
- For relapses 6 or more months after treatment, the original chemotherapy regimen may still be effective and can often be tried again.

Possible side effects of chemotherapy

Chemotherapy drugs work by attacking cells that are dividing quickly, which is why they work against cancer cells. But other cells in the body, such as those in the bone marrow (where new blood cells are made), the lining of the mouth and intestines, and the hair follicles, also divide quickly. These cells are also likely to be affected by chemotherapy, which can lead to side effects.

The side effects of chemotherapy depend on the type and dose of drugs given and the length of time they are taken. These are some possible side effects:

- hair loss
- mouth sores
- loss of appetite

- nausea and vomiting
- diarrhea or constipation
- increased chance of infections (because of low white blood cell counts)
- easy bruising or bleeding (because of low blood platelet counts)
- fatigue (because of low red blood cell counts)

These side effects are usually short-term and go away after treatment is finished. There are often ways to lessen these side effects. For example, there are drugs that can help prevent or reduce nausea and vomiting.

Some side effects can be longer-lasting. For example, drugs such as cisplatin, vinorelbine, docetaxel, or paclitaxel can damage nerves. This nerve damage can lead to symptoms, particularly in the hands and feet, such as pain, burning or tingling sensations, sensitivity to cold or heat, and weakness. This is called peripheral neuropathy. In most cases, peripheral neuropathy goes away once treatment is stopped, but it may be longer lasting in some people. For more information, visit our Web site at **cancer.org** or call **800-227-2345** and request the document *Peripheral Neuropathy Caused by Chemotherapy*. Also, cisplatin can cause kidney damage (called nephropathy). To help prevent this side effect, doctors increase intravenous fluids before and after each dose of the drug is given.

You should report any side effects you notice to your cancer care team so that they can be treated promptly. In some cases, the doses of the chemo-therapy drugs may need to be reduced, or treatment may need to be delayed or stopped to prevent side effects from getting worse.

For more information about chemotherapy, visit our Web site at **cancer.org** or call **800-227-2345** and request the document *Understanding Chemo-therapy: A Guide for Patients and Families.*

Treatment Choices by Stage for Small Cell Lung Cancer

As mentioned previously, for practical reasons, small cell lung cancer (SCLC) is usually staged as either limited stage or extensive stage. In most cases, SCLC has already metastasized by the time it is found—even if the metastasis is not seen on x-rays or other imaging tests—so it usually can-not be treated by surgery alone. If you are healthy enough, you will probably receive chemotherapy, regardless of the stage of your disease.

If you smoke, one of the most important things you can do to prepare for treatment is to try to quit. Studies have shown that patients who stop smoking after a diagnosis of lung cancer tend to have better outcomes than those who don't.

Limited stage small cell lung cancer
If you have only one nodule in your lung with no evidence of cancer elsewhere and you are in fairly good health, your doctors may recommend sur-gery to remove the tumor and the nearby lymph nodes. This would be followed by chemotherapy. Radiation to the chest is usually recommended if

cancer is found in the removed lymph nodes. The radiation is often given at the same time as the chemotherapy. Although this combination increases the side effects of treatment, it appears to be more effective than giving one treatment after the other. If you already have severe lung disease (in addition to your cancer) or other serious health problems, radiation therapy may not be an option for you.

If the cancer is larger, is in several places in the lung, or is found in the lymph nodes, surgery is not usually an option. The standard treatment for people who are otherwise in good health is chemotherapy plus radiation (given at the same time). People given these treatments together generally live longer and have a better chance of cure, but this treatment combination is often hard to take. If you have lung problems or other major health problems, chemotherapy may be given alone.

If no preventive measures are taken, the cancer will spread to the brain in about half of people with SCLC. For this reason, if your cancer has responded well to initial treatment, you may be given radiation therapy to the head (called prophylactic cranial irradiation, or PCI) to try to prevent metastasis to the brain. The radiation is usually given in lower doses than that given for treatment of known metastases. Still, some patients given PCI may experience side effects.

For most people treated with chemotherapy (with or without radiation) for limited stage SCLC, their tumors will shrink significantly. In about half of these people, the cancer will shrink to the point where it can no longer be seen on imaging tests. For most people, however, the cancer will return at some point.

Clinical trials of new chemotherapy drugs and combinations and other new treatments are being done to improve current treatment results. Because these cancers are hard to cure, a clinical trial may be a good option for some people. If you think you might be interested in a clinical trial, talk to your doctor.

Extensive stage small cell lung cancer

If you have extensive stage SCLC and are in fairly good health, chemotherapy can often treat your symptoms and extend your life. In about 3 of 4 people with extensive stage small cell lung cancer, chemotherapy will cause tumors to shrink significantly. Unfortunately, the cancer will still return at some point in almost all people with extensive stage SCLC. If the cancer responds well to chemotherapy, prophylactic cranial irradiation may be used to prevent metastasis to the brain.

Because these cancers are hard to treat, clinical trials of new chemotherapy drugs and combinations and other new treatments may be a good option for some people. If you think you might be interested in a clinical trial, talk to your doctor.

Radiation therapy is sometimes used to help shrink tumors and control symptoms, such as if cancer growth within the lungs is causing shortness of breath or bleeding. Other types of treatment, such as laser surgery, can sometimes be helpful in these situations. Radiation therapy can also be used to relieve symptoms if the cancer has spread to the bones or brain.

If your general health is poor, chemotherapy may not be an option for you. In this case, your doctor may select a treatment plan based on your individual situation. If you are too ill to undergo chemotherapy, the best plan may be to have supportive care. This would include treatment of any pain, breathing problems, or other symptoms.

Cancer that Progresses or Recurs After Treatment

If the cancer continues to grow during treatment or comes back after initial treatment, any further treatment will depend on the extent of the cancer, what treatments have been used, and the person's health and desire for further treatment. It is always important to understand the goal of any treatment before it starts—whether to try to cure the cancer, to slow its growth, or to help relieve symptoms— as well as the likelihood of benefits and risks.

If a cancer continues to grow during chemotherapy, another type of chemotherapy may be tried, although it may be less likely to be effective. For cancers that come back after initial treatment, the choice of chemotherapy drugs may depend on how long the cancer was in **remission**.

At some point, it may become clear that standard treatments are no longer controlling the cancer. If you want to continue anti-cancer treatment, you might think about taking part in a clinical trial of newer lung cancer treatments. Although clinical trials are not always the best option for every person, they may benefit you, as well as future patients.

Even if your cancer cannot be cured, you should strive to be as free of symptoms as possible. If curative treatment is not an option, treatment aimed at specific sites can often relieve symptoms and may even slow the spread of the disease. Symptoms caused by cancer in the airways—such as shortness of breath or coughing up blood—can often be treated effectively with radiation therapy, laser therapy, or other local treatments. Radiation therapy can be used to help control metastasis in the brain or relieve pain if cancer has spread to the bones.

Many people with lung cancer are concerned about pain. If the cancer grows near certain nerves, it can sometimes cause pain, but this can almost always be treated effectively with pain medicines. Sometimes radiation therapy or other treatments can be helpful. It is important that you talk to your doctor and take advantage of these treatment options.

Deciding on the right time to stop treatment aimed at curing the cancer and start focusing on care that relieves symptoms is never easy. Good communication with doctors, nurses, family, friends, and clergy can often help people facing this situation.

Additional Treatment Options to Consider

Clinical Trials

You probably have had to make many decisions since being told you have cancer. One of the most important decisions you will make is deciding which treatment is best for you. Maybe someone on your health care team has mentioned a **clinical trial** to you, or you may have heard about clinical trials being done for your type of cancer. Clinical trials are one way to get state-of-the art cancer care. Still, they are not right for everyone.

Here we will give you a brief overview of clinical trials. Talking to your health care team, your family, and your friends can help you make the best treatment choices.

Clinical trials are carefully controlled research studies that are done with patients. These studies test whether a new treatment is safe and how well it works in patients, or they may test new ways to diagnose or prevent a disease. Clinical trials have led to many advances in cancer prevention, diagnosis, and treatment.

Clinical trials are done to get a closer look at promising new treatments or procedures in patients. A clinical trial is undertaken only when there is good reason to believe that the treatment, test, or procedure being studied may be better than the one already being used. Treatments used in clinical trials are often found to have real benefits and may go on to become tomorrow's standard treatment.

Clinical trials can focus on many things:

- new uses of drugs that are already approved by the U.S. Food and Drug Administration (FDA)
- new drugs that have not yet been approved by the FDA
- nondrug treatments (such as radiation therapy)
- medical procedures (such as types of surgery)
- herbs and vitamins
- tools to improve the ways medicines or diagnostic tests are used
- medicines or procedures to relieve symptoms or improve comfort
- combinations of treatments and procedures

Researchers conduct studies of new treatments to try to answer the following questions:

- Is the treatment helpful?
- What is the best way to give it?
- Does it work better than other treatments already available?
- What side effects does the treatment cause?
- Are there more or fewer side effects than the standard treatment used now?
- Do the benefits outweigh the side effects?
- In which patients is the treatment most likely to be helpful?

Clinical trials are usually conducted in distinct phases. Each phase is designed to answer certain questions. Knowing the phase of the clinical trial is important because it can give you some idea about how much is known about the treatment being studied. There are pros and cons to taking part in each phase of a clinical trial.

Phase 0 clinical trials

Even though phase 0 studies are done in humans, this type of study is not much like the other phases of clinical trials. It is included here because some cancer patients may be asked to take part in these kinds of studies in the future.

Phase 0 studies are exploratory studies that often use only a few small doses of a new drug in each patient. They test to find out whether the drug reaches the tumor, how the drug acts in the human body, and how cancer cells respond to the drug. The patients in these studies must have extra biopsies, scans, and blood samples. The biggest difference between phase 0 and the later phases of clinical trials is that there is no chance the patient will be helped by taking part in a phase 0 trial. Because drug doses are low, there is also less risk to the patient in phase 0 studies compared with phase I studies.

Phase 0 studies help researchers find out which drugs do not do what they are expected to do. If there are problems with the way the drug is absorbed or acts in the body, this should become clear very quickly in a phase 0 trial. This process may help avoid the delay and expense of finding out years later in phase II or even phase III clinical trials that the drug doesn't act as it was expected to based on laboratory studies.

Phase 0 studies are not yet being used widely, and there are some drugs for which they would not be helpful. Phase 0 studies are very small, mostly with fewer than 20 people. They are not a required part of testing a new drug, but are part of an effort to speed up and streamline the process.

Phase I clinical trials

The purpose of a phase I study is to find the safest way to give a new treatment to patients. The cancer care team closely watches patients for any harmful side effects.

For phase I studies, the drug has already been tested in laboratory and animal studies, but the side effects in patients are not fully known. Doctors start by giving very low doses of the drug to the first patients and increase the doses for later groups of patients until side effects appear or the desired effect is seen. Doctors are hoping to help the study patients, but the main purpose of a phase I trial is to test the safety of the drug.

Phase I clinical trials are often done in small groups of people with different cancers that have not responded to standard treatment or that recur after treatment. If a drug is found to be reasonably safe in phase I studies, it can be tested in a phase II clinical trial.

Phase II clinical trials

These studies are designed to see whether the drug is effective. Patients are given the most appropriate (safest) dose as determined from phase I studies. They are closely watched for an effect on the cancer. The cancer care team also looks for side effects. Phase II trials are often done in larger groups of patients with a specific cancer type that has not responded to standard treatment. If a drug is found to be effective in phase II studies, it can be tested in a phase III clinical trial.

Phase III clinical trials

Phase III studies involve large numbers of patients—most often those patients who have just received a diagnosis for a specific type of cancer. Phase III clinical trials may enroll thousands of patients. Often, these studies are **randomized**, which means that patients are randomly put in 1 of 2 (or more) groups. One group (called the **control group**) gets the standard, most accepted treatment. The other group(s) gets the new treatment(s) being studied. All patients in phase III studies are closely watched. The study will be stopped early if many patients experience side effects that are too severe or if one group has much better results than the others. Phase III clinical trials are needed before the FDA will approve a treatment for use by the general public.

Phase IV clinical trials

Once a drug has been approved by the FDA and is available for all patients, it is still studied in other clinical trials (sometimes referred to as phase IV studies). This way, more can be learned about short-term and long-term side effects and safety as the drug is used in larger numbers of patients with many types of diseases. Doctors can also learn more about how well the drug works and whether it might be helpful when used in other ways (such as in combination with other treatments).

What it is like to be in a clinical trial

If you participate in a clinical trial, you will have a team of cancer care experts taking care of you and watching your progress very carefully. Depending on the phase of the clinical trial, you may receive more attention (such as having more doctor visits and laboratory tests) than you would if you were treated outside of a clinical trial. Clinical trials are designed to pay close attention to you. However, there are some risks. No one involved in the study knows in advance whether the treatment will work or exactly what side effects will occur. That is what the study is designed to find out. While most side effects go away in time, some may be long-lasting or even life threatening. Keep in mind, though, that even standard treatments have side effects.

Deciding to enter a clinical trial

If you would like to take part in a clinical trial, you should begin by asking your doctor whether your clinic or hospital conducts clinical trials. There are requirements you must meet to take part in any clinical trial. But whether you enroll in a clinical trial is completely up to you. The doctors and nurses conducting the study will explain the study to you in detail. They will go over the possible risks and benefits and give you an **informed consent** form to read and sign. The form says that you understand the clinical trial and want to take part in it. Even after you read and sign the form and the clinical trial begins, you are free to leave the study at any time, for any reason. Taking part in a clinical trial does not keep you from getting any other medical care you may need.

To find out more about clinical trials, talk to your cancer care team. Here are some questions you might ask:

- Is there a clinical trial that I should take part in?
- What is the purpose of the study?
- How might this study be of benefit to me?
- What is likely to happen in my case with, or without, this new treatment?
- What kinds of tests and treatments does the study involve?
- What does this treatment do? Has it been used before?
- Will I know which treatment I receive?
- What are my other choices and their pros and cons?
- How could the study affect my daily life?
- What side effects can I expect from the study? Can the side effects be controlled?
- Will I have to stay in the hospital? If so, how often and for how long?

- Will the study cost me anything? Will any of the treatment be free?
- If I am harmed as a result of the research, what treatment would I be entitled to?
- What type of long-term follow-up care is part of the study?
- Has the treatment been used for other types of cancer?

How can I find out more about clinical trials that might be right for me?

The American Cancer Society offers a clinical trials matching service for use by patients, their family, or friends. You can reach this service at **800-303-5691** or on the Web at **http://clinicaltrials .cancer.org**.

Based on the information you give about your cancer type, stage, and previous treatments, this service can put together a list of clinical trials that match your medical needs. The service will also ask where you live and whether you are willing to travel so that it can look for a treatment center that you can get to. You can also get a list of current clinical trials by calling the National Cancer Institute's Cancer Information Service toll-free at **800-4-CANCER (800-422-6237)** or by visiting the NCI clinical trials Web site at **www.cancer .gov/clinicaltrials**.

For even more information on clinical trials, visit our Web site at **cancer.org** or call **800-227-2345** and request the document *Clinical Trials: What You Need to Know*.

Complementary and Alternative Treatments

When you have cancer, you are likely to hear about ways to treat your cancer or relieve symptoms that are different from standard medical treatments. These treatments can include vitamins, herbs, and special diets, or acupuncture and massage— among many others. You may have a lot of questions about these treatments. Talk to your doctor about any treatment you are considering. Here are some questions to ask:

- How do I know whether the treatment is safe?
- How do I know whether it works?
- Should I try one or more of these treatments?
- Will these treatments cause a problem with my standard medical treatment?
- What is the difference between complementary and alternative treatments?
- Where can I find out more about these treatments?

The terms can be confusing

Not everyone uses these terms the same way, so it can be confusing. The American Cancer Society uses **complementary medicine** to refer to medicines or treatments that are used *along with* your regular medical care. **Alternative medicine** is a treatment used *instead of* standard medical treatment.

Complementary treatments

Complementary treatment methods, for the most part, are not presented as cures for cancer. Most often, they are used to help you feel better. Some methods that can be used in a complementary way are meditation to reduce stress, acupuncture to relieve pain, or peppermint tea to relieve nausea. There are many others. Some of these methods are known to help and could add to your comfort and well-being, whereas others have not been tested. Some have been proven not to be helpful. A few have even been found harmful. There are many complementary methods that you can safely use with your medical treatment to help relieve symptoms or side effects, to ease pain, and to help you enjoy life more. For example, some people find methods such as aromatherapy, massage therapy, meditation, or yoga to be useful.

Alternative treatments

Alternative treatments are methods that are used instead of standard medical care. These treatments have not been proven to be safe and effective in clinical trials. Some of these treatments may even be dangerous or have life-threatening side effects. The biggest danger in most cases is that you may lose the chance to benefit from standard treatment. Delays or interruptions in your standard medical treatment may give the cancer more time to grow.

Deciding what to do

It is easy to see why people with cancer may consider alternative treatments. You want to do all you can to fight the cancer. Sometimes main-stream treatments such as chemotherapy can be hard to take, or they may no longer be working. Sometimes people suggest that their treatment can cure your cancer without having serious side effects, and it is normal to want to believe them. But the truth is that most nonstandard treatments have not been tested and proven to be effective for treating cancer.

As you consider your options, here are 3 important steps you can take:

- Talk to your doctor or nurse about any treatments you are thinking about using.
- Check the list of "red flags" below.
- Contact the American Cancer Society at **800-227-2345** to learn more about complementary and alternative treatments in general and to learn more about the specific treatments you are considering.

Red flags

You can use the following questions to spot treatments or methods to avoid. A "yes" answer to any one of these questions should raise a red flag.

- Does the treatment promise a cure?
- Are you told not to use standard medical treatment?
- Is the treatment or drug a "secret" that only certain people can give?
- Does the treatment require you to travel to another country?
- Do the promoters of the treatment attack the medical or scientific community?

The decision is yours

Decisions about how to treat or manage your cancer are always yours to make. If you are thinking about using a complementary or alternative method, be sure to learn about it and talk with your doctor about it. With reliable information and the support of your cancer care team, you may be able to safely use methods that can help you while avoiding those that could be harmful.

More Treatment Information

For more details on treatment options—including some that may not be addressed in this book—the National Cancer Institute (NCI) and the National Comprehensive Cancer Network (NCCN) are good sources of information. The NCI provides treatment guidelines via its telephone information center (800-4-CANCER) and its Web site (www.cancer.gov). The NCCN, made up of experts from many of the nation's leading cancer centers, develops cancer treatment guidelines for doctors to use when treating patients. These guidelines are available on the NCCN Web site (www.nccn.org). The NCCN also has patient versions of treatment guidelines for lung cancer, available at www.nccn.org.

Questions
to Ask

What Should You Ask Your Doctor About Lung Cancer?

It is important for you to have honest, open discussions with your cancer care team. They want to answer all of your questions, no matter how minor you might think they are. Here are some questions to consider:

- What kind of lung cancer do I have?
- Has my cancer spread beyond the primary site?
- What is the stage of my cancer, and what does that mean in my case?
- Are there other tests that need to be done before we can decide on treatment?
- Are there other doctors I need to see?
- How much experience do you have treating this type of cancer?
- What treatment choices do I have?
- What do you recommend and why?
- What is the goal of the treatment?
- What are the chances my cancer can be cured with these options?

- What risks or side effects are there to the treatments you suggest? How long are they likely to last?
- How quickly do we need to decide on a treatment plan?
- What should I do to be ready for treatment?
- How long will treatment last? What will it involve? Where will it be done?
- What would we do if the treatment doesn't work or the cancer recurs?
- What type of follow-up will I need after treatment?

Along with these sample questions, be sure to write down your own. For instance, you might want more information about recovery times so you can plan your work or activity schedule. Or you may want to ask about second opinions or about clinical trials for which you may qualify.

After Treatment

What Happens After Treatment for Lung Cancer?

Completing treatment can be both stressful and exciting. You may be relieved to finish treatment but find it difficult not to worry about cancer coming back. (When cancer comes back after treatment, it is called **recurrence**.) The fear of recurrence is very common among people who have had cancer. It may take some time for your fears to lessen and for you to have confidence in your own recovery. Even with no recurrence, people who have had cancer learn to live with some uncertainty. For more information on managing these feelings, contact your American Cancer Society at **800-227-2345** and request the document *Living With Uncertainty: The Fear of Cancer Recurrence*, or visit our Web site, **cancer.org**.

For some other people, the lung cancer may never go away completely. These people may get regular treatments with chemotherapy, radiation therapy, or other therapies to help keep the cancer in check. Learning to live with cancer as a chronic disease can be difficult and very stressful. This situation has its own type of uncertainty, but many people learn to live with cancer and continue to live full lives. For more information, contact the American Cancer Society at **800-227-2345** and request the document *When Cancer Doesn't Go Away*, or visit **cancer.org**.

Follow-up Care

If you have completed treatment, your doctors will still want to monitor you closely. It is very important to go to all of your follow-up appointments. In people with no signs of cancer remaining, most doctors recommend follow-up visits and CT scans every 4 to 6 months for the first 2 years after treatment, with yearly visits and CT scans from then on as needed.

Follow-up care is needed to check for cancer recurrence, metastasis, and possible side effects of certain treatments. Almost any cancer treatment can have side effects. Some may last for a few weeks to several months, but others can last the rest of your life. Don't hesitate to tell your cancer care team about any symptoms or side effects that bother you so they can help you manage them. These visits are the time for you to talk to your cancer care team about any changes or problems you notice and any questions or concerns you have. During these visits, your doctors will ask questions and may do examinations and laboratory tests or imaging tests, such as x-rays or CT scans.

If cancer does recur, treatment will depend on the location of the cancer and what treatments you've already had. The recommended treatment may be surgery, radiation therapy, chemotherapy, targeted therapy, or some combination of these. For more information on how recurrent cancer is treated, see the sections on treatment choices by cancer type and stage (beginning on pages 100 and 121). For more general information on dealing with a recurrence, contact your American Cancer Society at **800-227-2345** and request the document *When Your Cancer Comes Back: Cancer Recurrence*, or visit our Web site, **cancer.org**.

Seeing a New Doctor

At some point after your cancer diagnosis and treatment, you may find yourself seeing a new doctor, a doctor who knows nothing about your medical history. It is important that you be able to give your new doctor the details of your cancer diagnosis and treatment. Make sure you have the following information handy:

- a copy of your pathology report(s) from any biopsies or surgeries
- a copy of your operative report(s) if you had surgery
- if you were hospitalized, a copy of the discharge summary that doctors prepare when patients are sent home
- if you had radiation therapy, a summary of the type and dose of radiation and when and where it was given

- If you had chemotherapy or targeted therapies, a list of the drugs, dosages, and when you took them

It is very important to keep health insurance. Tests and doctor visits are expensive, and even though no one wants to think about a cancer recurrence, it is a possibility.

Lifestyle Changes to Consider During and After Treatment

You cannot change the fact that you have had cancer. What you can change is how you live the rest of your life—making choices to help you stay healthy and feel as well as you can. This can be a time to look at your life in new ways. Maybe you are thinking about how to improve your health over the long term. Some people even start making changes to improve their health while they are going through cancer treatment.

Make Healthier Choices

For many people, a cancer diagnosis helps them focus on their health in ways they may not have thought much about in the past. Are there things you could do to improve your health? Maybe you could try to eat better or get more exercise. Maybe you could cut down on alcohol or give up tobacco. Even things like keeping your stress level under control may help. Now is a good time to think about making changes that can have positive effects for the rest of your life. You will feel better and be healthier.

You can start by working on the things that worry you the most. Get help with changes that are harder for you. For instance, if you smoke, one of the most important things you can do to improve your health is to quit. Studies have shown that people who stop smoking after a lung cancer diagnosis have better outcomes than those who continue to smoke. If you are thinking about quitting smoking and need help, call the American Cancer Society at **800-227-2345** or visit our Web site, **cancer.org**.

Diet and nutrition

Eating right can be difficult for anyone, but it can get even tougher during and after cancer treatment. Treatment may change your sense of taste. Nausea can be a problem. You may lose your appetite and lose weight when you don't want to. Or you may have gained weight that you cannot seem to lose. All of these things can be very frustrating.

If treatment caused weight changes or problems with eating, do the best you can and keep in mind that these problems usually get better over time. You may find that it helps to eat small portions every 2 to 3 hours until you feel better. You may also want to ask your cancer care team about seeing a registered dietitian, an expert in nutrition who can give you ideas on how to deal with treatment side effects.

One of the best things you can do after cancer treatment is put healthy eating habits into place. You may be surprised at the long-term benefits of some simple changes, like increasing the variety of healthy foods you eat. Getting to and staying at a healthy weight, eating a healthy diet, and limiting your alcohol intake may lower your risk for some other cancers, as well as having many other health benefits.

Rest, fatigue, work, and exercise

Fatigue, or extreme tiredness, is very common in people treated for cancer. Fatigue is not an ordinary tiredness but a bone-weary exhaustion that does not improve with rest. For some people, fatigue can last a long time after treatment and can make it hard to exercise and do other things they want to do. Exercise, however, can actually help reduce fatigue. Studies have shown that people who follow an exercise program tailored to their personal needs feel better physically and emotionally and can cope better.

If you were not able to be very active during treatment, it is normal for your fitness, endurance, and muscle strength to decline. Any plan for physical activity should fit your situation. An older person who has never exercised will not be able to take on the same amount of exercise as a 20-year-old who is accustomed to playing tennis twice a week. If you have not exercised in a few years, you will have to start slowly—maybe just by taking short walks.

Talk with your health care team before starting any exercise program. Get their opinion about your exercise plans. Then, recruit a family member or friend to join you. Having an exercise buddy will give you the extra boost of support you need to keep you going when you may not feel as motivated.

If you are very tired, you will need to balance activity with rest. It is important that you rest when you need to. It can be hard for people who are used to working all day or taking care of a household to allow themselves to rest, but it is crucial. Listen to your body and rest when you need to.

Keep in mind exercise can improve your physical and emotional health in several ways:

- It improves your cardiovascular (heart and circulation) fitness.
- Along with a good diet, it will help you get to and stay at a healthy weight.
- It strengthens your muscles.
- It reduces fatigue and helps you have more energy.
- It can help lower anxiety and depression.
- It makes you feel happier.
- It helps you feel better about yourself.

Long term, we know that exercise plays a role in lowering the risk of some cancers. The American Cancer Society, in its guidelines on physical activity for cancer prevention, recommends that adults take part in at least 30 minutes of moderate to vigorous physical activity, above usual activities, on 5 or more days of the week; 45 to 60 minutes of intentional physical activity is preferable.

Can I lower my risk of the cancer progressing or coming back?

Most people want to know whether there are specific lifestyle changes they can make to reduce their risk of cancer progressing or coming back. Unfortunately, for most cancers there is little solid evidence to guide people. This does not mean that nothing will help—rather, this is an area that has not been well studied. Most studies have looked at the effect of lifestyle changes on preventing cancer in the first place, not slowing it down or preventing it from coming back.

However, there are some steps people can take that might help them live longer or reduce the risk of lung cancer recurring.

Quitting smoking: If you smoke, quitting is important. It has been shown to help improve outcomes and reduce the risk of recurrence, especially in people with early-stage lung cancer. Of course, quitting smoking may have other health benefits as well, including lowering the risk of some other cancers. If you need help quitting, talk to your doctor or call the American Cancer Society at **800-227-2345**.

Diet and nutrition: Possible links between diet and lung cancer progression or recurrence are much less clear. As noted earlier, some studies have suggested that diets high in fruits and vegetables might help prevent lung cancer from developing in the first place, but this theory has not been studied in people who already have lung cancer. Some early studies have suggested that people with early-stage lung cancer who have higher vitamin D levels might have better outcomes, but more research is needed. On the other hand, studies have found that beta carotene supplements may actually increase the risk of lung cancer in smokers. Because of the lack of data in this area, it's important to talk with your health care team before making any major dietary changes (including taking any supplements) to try to improve your prognosis.

Your Emotional Health

During and after treatment, you may find yourself overcome with many emotions. This is common. You may have been going through so much during treatment that you could focus only on getting through each day. Now it may feel like other issues are catching up with you.

You may find yourself thinking about death and dying. You may be more aware of the effect the cancer has had on your family, friends, and career. You may reexamine your relationships with those around you. Unexpected issues may also cause concern. For instance, as you feel better and have fewer doctor visits, you will see your health care team less often and have more time on your hands. These changes can make some people anxious.

Almost everyone who has been through cancer can benefit from getting some type of support. You need people you can turn to for strength and comfort. Support can come in many forms: family, friends, counselors, cancer support groups, church or spiritual groups, or online support communities. What's best for you depends on your situation and personality. Some people feel safe in peer-support groups or education groups. Others would rather talk in an informal setting, such as church. Others feel more at ease talking one-on-one with a trusted friend or counselor. Whatever your source of strength or comfort, make sure you have a place to go with your concerns.

The cancer journey can feel very lonely. It is not necessary or good for you to try to deal with everything on your own. In addition, your friends and family may feel shut out if you do not include them. Allow them—and anyone else you feel may be able to help—to be there for you. If you are not sure who can help, call your American Cancer Society at **800-227-2345** to find out about nearby groups or other resources that can help you.

What Happens If Treatment Is No Longer Working?

If cancer continues to grow or return after one kind of treatment, it is often possible to try another treatment plan that might still cure the cancer or shrink the tumors enough to help you live longer and feel better. When a person has tried many different treatments, however, and the cancer has not gotten better, the cancer tends to become resistant to all treatment. If this happens, it is important to weigh the possible limited benefits of a new treatment against the possible disadvantages, including treatment side effects.

This is likely to be the hardest part of your battle with cancer—when you have been through many medical treatments and nothing is working anymore. Although your doctor may offer you new treatment options, at some point you may need to consider that further treatment is not likely to improve your health or change your outcome or survival.

If you want to continue treatment for as long as you can, you need to consider whether treatment will have any benefit and how this compares to the possible risks and side effects. In many cases, your doctor can estimate how likely it is the cancer will respond to treatment you are considering. For instance, the doctor may say that more treatment might have about a 1 in 100 chance of working. Whatever your decision, it is important to think about and understand the reasons behind your choice.

No matter what you decide to do, you need to feel as good as you can. Make sure you are asking for and getting treatment for any symptoms you have, such as nausea or pain. This type of treatment is called **palliative care**.

Palliative care helps relieve symptoms but is not expected to cure the disease. The main purpose of palliative care is to improve the quality of your life, or help you feel as good as you can for as long as you can. Sometimes, this means using drugs to help with such symptoms as pain or nausea. Sometimes, the treatments used to control symptoms are the same as those used to treat cancer. For instance, radiation might be used to help relieve bone pain caused by cancer that has spread to the bones. Chemotherapy might be used to help shrink a tumor and keep it from blocking the bowels. But this is not the same as treatment to try to cure the cancer.

At some point, you may benefit from **hospice** care. This is special care that treats the person rather than the disease; it focuses on quality rather than length of life. Most of the time, hospice care is given at home. While getting hospice care may mean the end of treatments such as chemotherapy and radiation, it does not mean you can't have treatment for the problems caused by your cancer or other health conditions. In hospice, the focus of your care is on living life as fully as possible and feeling as well as you can. For more information on hospice care, contact the American Cancer Society at **800-227-2345** and request the document *Hospice Care*, or visit our Web site, **cancer.org**.

Staying hopeful is important, too. Your hope for a cure may not be as bright, but there is still hope for good times with family and friends— times that are filled with happiness and meaning. Pausing at this time in your cancer treatment gives you a chance to refocus on the most important things in your life. Now is the time to do the things you have always wanted to do and to stop doing things you no longer want to do. Though cancer may be beyond your control, there are still choices you can make.

Latest
Research

What's New in Lung Cancer Research and Treatment?

Lung cancer research is currently being done in medical centers throughout the world. Progress in prevention, early detection, and treatment based on current research is expected to save many thousands of lives each year.

Prevention

Tobacco

At this time, many researchers believe that prevention offers the greatest opportunity to fight lung cancer. Although decades have passed since the link between smoking and lung cancer was clearly identified, scientists estimate that smoking is still responsible for about 87% of lung cancer deaths. Research is continuing in several areas related to smoking:

- ways to help people quit smoking through counseling, nicotine replacement, and medicines

- ways to convince young people to never start smoking
- inherited differences in genes that may make some people much more likely to get lung cancer if they smoke or are exposed to other's smoke

Diet, nutrition, and medicines

Although researchers are looking for ways to use vitamins or medicines to prevent lung cancer in people at high risk, so far none have been shown conclusively to reduce risk. Some studies have suggested that a diet high in fruits and vegetables may offer some protection against lung cancer, but more research is needed. For now, most researchers think that simply following the American Cancer Society dietary recommendations (such as maintaining a healthy weight and eating at least 5 servings of fruits and vegetables each day) may be the best strategy for prevention.

Early Detection

In the past, large studies were done to determine whether routine chest x-rays and sputum cytology testing could save lives. Most researchers concluded that these tests did not find lung cancers early enough to significantly lower the risk of death from the disease. However, there is some disagreement among researchers, and the debate continues.

As mentioned on page 27, a large clinical trial called the National Lung Screening Trial (NLST) recently found that spiral CT scanning in people at high risk for lung cancer because of a history of smoking lowered the risk of death from lung cancer when compared to chest x-rays. The implications of this finding should become more apparent in the near future.

Another approach to early detection uses newer, more sensitive tests to look for cancer cells in sputum samples. Researchers have recently found changes in the DNA of lung cancer cells. Current studies are looking at new diagnostic tests that specifically recognize these DNA changes to see whether this approach could be useful in finding lung cancers at an earlier stage.

Diagnosis

Fluorescence bronchoscopy

Known as **fluorescence bronchoscopy** or auto-fluorescence bronchoscopy, this technique may help doctors find lung cancers earlier, when they could be easier to treat. For this test, the doctor inserts a bronchoscope through the mouth or nose and into the lungs. The end of the bronchoscope has a special fluorescent light on it (instead of a normal, white light). The fluorescent light causes abnormal areas in the airways to show up in a different color than healthy tissues, helping doctors find abnormal tissues sooner. Some cancer centers now use this technique to look for early-stage lung cancers, especially if no obvious tumors can be seen with normal bronchoscopy.

Virtual bronchoscopy

Virtual bronchoscopy uses CT scans to create detailed 3-dimensional pictures of the airways in the lungs. The images can be viewed as if the doctor were actually using a bronchoscope. Virtual bronchoscopy has some possible advantages over standard bronchoscopy. First, it is noninvasive and does not require anesthesia. It also allows doctors to see airways that might not be visible with standard bronchoscopy, such as those being blocked by a tumor. But it has some drawbacks as well. For example, it does not show color changes in the airways that could indicate abnormalities. It also does not allow doctors to take samples of suspicious areas, as bronchoscopy does. Still, it can be a useful tool in some situations, such as in people who are too sick for standard bronchoscopy. This test will likely become more widely available as technology improves.

Treatment

Chemotherapy

New combinations: Many clinical trials are comparing the effectiveness of newer combinations of chemotherapy drugs. These studies are also providing information about reducing side effects, especially in patients who are older and have other health problems. Doctors are also studying better ways to combine chemotherapy with radiation therapy and other treatments.

Predicting the effectiveness of chemotherapy: Doctors know that adjuvant chemotherapy may be more helpful for some people with early (stage I or II) non–small cell lung cancer. Determining which patients will benefit, however, is not easy. In early studies, newer laboratory tests looking at patterns of certain genes in cancer cells have shown promise in predicting which people might benefit most. Larger studies of these tests are now under way.

Other laboratory tests may help predict whether some types of non–small cell lung cancer will respond to particular chemotherapy drugs. For example, studies have found that tumors with high levels of the protein ERCC1 are less likely to respond to chemotherapy that includes cisplatin or carboplatin, whereas tumors with high levels of the protein RRM1 seem less likely to respond to chemotherapy that includes gemcitabine. Some doctors are now testing for these markers as a way to help guide the choice of treatment.

Maintenance chemotherapy: For people with advanced non–small cell lung cancer who can tolerate chemotherapy, combinations of 2 drugs are typically given for about 4 to 6 cycles. Doctors often do not give additional chemotherapy beyond that initial regimen unless the cancer starts growing again. In the case of cancers that have not progressed, recent studies have found that continuing treatment beyond the 4 to 6 cycles with a single drug—either a chemotherapy drug such as pemetrexed or a targeted drug such as erlotinib—may help some people live longer. This is known as maintenance therapy. A possible downside to maintenance therapy is that people may not get a break from side effects of chemotherapy. Some doctors now recommend maintenance therapy, while others await further research on this topic.

Targeted therapies

Researchers are learning more about the mechanisms of lung cancer cells that control their growth and spread. This information is being used to develop new targeted therapies. These drugs work differently from standard chemotherapy drugs. They often have different (and less severe) side effects. Many of these treatments are already being tested in clinical trials to see whether they can help people with advanced lung cancer live longer or help relieve their symptoms.

Some of the other targeted drugs in late-stage clinical trials include vadimezan (DMXAA, ASA404), afatinib (BIBW 2992), and motesanib (AMG 706). Some targeted drugs already approved for use against other types of cancer, such as sorafenib (Nexavar) and sunitinib (Sutent), are also being tested for use against non–small cell lung cancer.

Researchers are also working on laboratory tests to help predict which patients will benefit from which drugs. Studies have found that some people do not benefit from certain targeted therapies, whereas others are more likely to have their tumors shrink significantly. For example, a test that finds changes in the *EGFR* gene can indicate whether a person's lung cancer is likely to respond to treatment with erlotinib (Tarceva), an EGFR inhibitor.

Similar gene tests are now being studied. Predicting who could benefit from specific treatments could save some people from trying treatments that are unlikely to work and likely to cause side effects.

Anti-angiogenesis drugs: For cancers to grow, new blood vessels must develop to nourish the cancer cells within tumors. This process is called angiogenesis. New drugs that inhibit angiogenesis are being studied as treatments for small cell lung cancer. Some have already been successfully used for other cancer types. For example, a drug called bevacizumab (Avastin) has been shown to help patients with some types of non–small cell lung cancer and is now being tested in small cell lung cancer. Other drugs already approved for use against other types of cancer, such as sunitinib (Sutent) and sorafenib (Nexavar), are also being tested for use against small cell lung cancer.

Vaccines: Several types of vaccines for boosting the body's immune response against lung cancer cells are being tested in clinical trials. Unlike vaccines against such infections as measles or mumps, these vaccines are designed to help treat, not prevent, lung cancer. One possible advantage of vaccines is that they seem to have very limited side effects, so they might be useful in people who can't tolerate other treatments.

Some vaccines are made up of lung cancer cells that have been grown in the laboratory, or even of cell components, such as parts of proteins commonly found on cancer cells. For example, the MUC1 protein is found on some lung cancer cells. A vaccine called TG4010 causes the immune system to react against that protein. A recent study compared the effectiveness of combining the vaccine with chemotherapy to use of the same chemotherapy alone in patients with advanced lung cancer. In the group that got the vaccine, patients' cancers were more likely to shrink or stop growing than in the group that got only chemotherapy. More studies are planned to see whether the vaccine will actually help patients live longer.

L-BLP25 (Stimuvax) is another vaccine that targets the MUC1 protein. It is made up of a protein (MUC1) encased in a liposome (a fat droplet) to make it more effective. A small study of people with advanced NSCLC suggested it may improve survival time. Larger studies are being done to try to confirm this finding.

At this time, vaccines are only available in clinical trials.

Talactoferrin (TLF): This protein is a genetically engineered form of the human protein lactoferrin, which is normally found in body secretions such as breast milk, tears, and saliva. In studies, TLF has been shown to stimulate the immune system. It seems to have anti-infective and anti-inflammatory properties, as well as anti-tumor activity. In a recent study of people with advanced lung cancer whose cancers had grown despite previous chemotherapy, the group that received TLF lived longer than the group that received the placebo (sugar pill). There were few side effects related to treatment. A larger study is planned.

Resources

Additional Resources

The American Cancer Society can address any cancer-related topic. If you have questions, please call us at **800-227-2345**, 24 hours a day.

More Information from Your American Cancer Society

The following related materials may be ordered through our toll-free number: **800-227-2345**.

Spanish language versions of some of these documents are also available.

After Diagnosis: A Guide for Patients and Families

Asbestos

Caring for the Patient With Cancer at Home: A Guide for Patients and Families

Guide to Quitting Smoking

Lasers in Cancer Treatment

Living With Uncertainty: The Fear of Cancer Recurrence

Pain Control: A Guide for Those With Cancer and Their Loved Ones

Peripheral Neuropathy Caused by Chemotherapy

Photodynamic Therapy

Questions About Smoking, Tobacco, and Health

Radon

Skin Changes Caused by Targeted Therapies

Surgery

Understanding Chemotherapy: A Guide for Patients and Families

Understanding Radiation Therapy: A Guide for Patients and Families

When Your Cancer Comes Back: Cancer Recurrence

National Organizations and Web sites*

In addition to the American Cancer Society, the following other sources of patient information and support are available:

American Lung Association
Toll-free number: 800-586-4872 (800-LUNGUSA)
Internet address: www.lungusa.org

Lungcancer.org
Toll-free number: 800-813-4673 (800-813-HOPE)
Internet address: www.lungcancer.org

Lung Cancer Alliance
Toll-free number: 800-298-2436
Internet address: www.lungcanceralliance.org

National Cancer Institute
Toll-free number: 800-422-6237 (800-4-CANCER)
Internet address: www.cancer.gov

References

Alberg AJ, Brock MV, Stuart JM. Epidemiology of lung cancer: looking to the future. *J Clin Oncol.* 2005;23(14):3175–3185.

American Cancer Society

American Cancer Society. *Cancer Facts & Figures 2012.* Atlanta, GA: American Cancer Society; 2012.

American Cancer Society. *Cancer Facts & Figures for African Americans 2009–2010.* Atlanta, GA: American Cancer Society; 2009.

American Joint Committee on Cancer. Lung. *AJCC Cancer Staging Manual.* 7th ed. New York: Springer. 2010:253–266.

Bach PB, Silvestri GA, Hanger M, Jett JR; American College of Chest Physicians. Screening for lung cancer: ACCP evidence-based clinical practice guidelines (2nd edition). *Chest.* 2007;132(3 Suppl):69S–77S.

Bailey-Wilson JE, Amos CI, Pinney SM, Petersen GM, de Andrade M, Wiest JS, Fain P, Schwartz AG, You M, Franklin W, Klein C, Gazdar A, Rothschild H, Mandal D, Coons T, Slusser J, Lee J, Gaba C, Kupert E, Perez A, Zhou X, Zeng D, Liu Q, Zhang Q, Seminara D, Minna J, Anderson MW. A major lung cancer susceptibility locus maps to chromosome 6q23–25. *Am J Hum Genet.* 2004;75(3):460–474. Epub 2004 Jul 21.

Butts C, Murray N, Maksymiuk A, Goss G, Marshall E, Soulières D, Cormier Y, Ellis P, Price A, Sawhney R, Davis M, Mansi J, Smith C, Vergidis D, Ellis P, MacNeil M, Palmer M. Randomized phase IIB trial of BLP25 liposome vaccine in stage IIIB and IV non-small-cell lung cancer. *J Clin Oncol* 2005;23(27):6674–6681.

Ciuleanu T, Brodowicz T, Zielinski C, Kim JH, Krzakowski M, Laack E, Wu YL, Bover I, Begbie S, Tzekova V, Cucevic B, Pereira JR, Yang SH, Madhavan J, Sugarman KP, Peterson P, John WJ, Krejcy K, Belani CP. Maintenance pemetrexed plus best supportive care versus placebo plus best supportive care for non-small-cell lung cancer: a randomised, double-blind, phase 3 study. *Lancet.* 2009;374(9699):1432–1440. Epub 2009 Sep 18.

Cohen AJ, Anderson HR, Ostro B, Pandey KD, Krzyzanowski M, Künzli N, Gutschmidt K, Pope A, Romieu I, Samet JM, Smith K. The global burden of disease due to outdoor air pollution. *J Toxicol Environ Health A.* 2005;68(13–14):1301–1307.

Groome PA, Bolejack V, Crowley JJ, Kennedy C, Krasnik M, Sobin LH, Goldstraw P; IASLC International Staging Committee; Cancer Research and Biostatistics; Observers to the Committee; Participating Institutions. The IASLC Lung Cancer Staging Project: validation of the proposals for revision of the T, N, and M descriptors and consequent stage groupings in the forthcoming (seventh) edition of the TNM classification of malignant tumours. *J Thorac Oncol.* 2007;2(8):694–705.

Howlader N, Noone AM, Krapcho M, Neyman N, Aminou R, Waldron W, Altekruse SF, Kosary CL, Ruhl J, Tatalovich Z, Cho H, Mariotto A, Eisner MP, Lewis DR, Chen HS, Feuer EJ, Cronin KA, Edwards BK (eds). SEER Cancer Statistics Review, 1975–2008, National Cancer Institute. Bethesda, MD. http://seer.cancer.gov/csr/1975_2009_pops09/, based on November 2010 SEER data submission, posted to the SEER Web site, 2011.

Jackman DM, Johnson BE. Small-cell lung cancer. *Lancet.* 2005;366(9494):1385–1396.

Johnson DH, Blot WJ, Carbone DP, et al. Cancer of the lung: non-small cell lung cancer and small cell lung cancer. In: Abeloff MD, Armitage JO, Niederhuber JE, Kastan MB, McKenna WG, eds. *Abeloff's Clinical Oncology.* 4th ed. Philadelphia, PA: Elsevier; 2008:1307–1366.

Kaufman EL, Jacobson JS, Hershman DL, Desai M, Neugut AI. Effect of breast cancer radiotherapy and cigarette smoking on risk of second primary lung cancer. *J Clin Oncol.* 2008;26(3):392–398.

Krug LM, Kris MG, Rosenzweig K, Travis WD. Small cell and other neuroendocrine tumors of the lung. In: DeVita VT, Lawrence TS, Rosenberg SA, eds. *DeVita, Hellman, and Rosenberg's Cancer: Principles and Practice of Oncology.* 8th ed. Philadelphia, PA: Lippincott Williams & Wilkins; 2008:946–971.

Kwak EL, Bang YJ, Camidge DR, Shaw AT, Solomon B, Maki RG, Ou SH, Dezube BJ, Jänne PA, Costa DB, Varella-Garcia M, Kim WH, Lynch TJ, Fidias P, Stubbs H, Engelman JA, Sequist LV, Tan W, Gandhi L, Mino-Kenudson M, Wei GC, Shreeve SM, Ratain MJ, Settleman J, Christensen JG, Haber DA, Wilner K, Salgia R, Shapiro GI, Clark JW, Iafrate AJ. Anaplastic lymphoma kinase inhibition in non-small cell lung cancer. *New Engl J Med.* 2010;363(18):1693–1703.

Masters GA. Clinical presentation of small cell lung cancer. In: Pass HI, Carbone DP, Johnson DH, Minna JD, Scagliotti GV, Turrisi AT, eds. *Principles and Practice of Lung Cancer.* 4th ed. Philadelphia, PA: Lippincott Williams & Wilkins. 2010:341–351.

National Cancer Institute. Physician Data Query (PDQ). Non-Small Cell Lung Cancer Treatment. 2011. National Cancer Institute Web site. www.cancer.gov/cancertopics/pdq/treatment/non-small-cell-lung/healthprofessional. Accessed January 23, 2012.

National Cancer Institute. Physician Data Query (PDQ). Small Cell Lung Cancer Treatment. 2010. National Cancer Institute Web site. www.cancer.gov/cancertopics/pdq/treatment/small-cell-lung/healthprofessional. Accessed November 1, 2010.

National Comprehensive Cancer Network. NCCN Clinical Practice Guidelines in Oncology: Non-Small Cell Lung Cancer. V.2.2012. National

Comprehensive Cancer Network Web site. www
.nccn.org/professionals/physician_gls/PDF/nscl.pdf.
Accessed January 13, 2012.

National Comprehensive Cancer Network. NCCN
Clinical Practice Guidelines in Oncology: Small Cell
Lung Cancer. V.1.2011. National Comprehensive
Cancer Network Web site. www.nccn.org/
professionals/physician_gls/PDF/sclc.pdf. Accessed
November 1, 2010.

National Lung Screening Trial Research Team, Aberle
DR, Adams AM, Berg CD, Black WC, Clapp JD,
Fagerstrom RM, Gareen IF, Gatsonis C, Marcus
PM, Sicks JD. Reduced lung-cancer mortality with
low-dose computed tomographic screening. *N Engl
J Med.* 2011;365(5):395–409. Epub 2011 Jun 29.
Epub 2011 Jun 29.

Obedian E, Fischer DB, Haffty BG. Second malignancies
after treatment of early-stage breast cancer:
lumpectomy and radiation therapy versus
mastectomy. *J Clin Oncol.* 2000;18(12):2406–2412.

Parikh PM, Vaid A, Advani SH, Digumarti R,
Madhavan J, Nag S, Bapna A, Sekhon JS, Patil S,
Ismail PM, Wang Y, Varadhachary A, Zhu J, Malik
R. Randomized, double-blind, placebo-controlled
phase II study of single-agent oral talactoferrin
in patients with locally advanced or metastatic
non-small-cell lung cancer that progressed after
chemotherapy. *J Clin Oncol.* 2011;29(31):4129–
4136. Epub 2011 Oct 3.

Parsons A, Daley A, Begh R, Aveyard P. Influence of
smoking cessation after diagnosis of early stage
lung cancer on prognosis: systematic review of
observational studies with meta-analysis. *BMJ.*
2010;340:b5569.

Pletcher MJ, Vittinghoff E, Kalhan R, Richman J, Safford
M, Sidney S, Lin F, Kertesz S. Association between

marijuana exposure and pulmonary function over 20 years. *JAMA.* 2012;307(2):173–181.

Posther KE, Harpole DH Jr. The surgical management of lung cancer. *Cancer Invest.* 2006;24(1):56–67.

Price T, Nichols F. Surgical management of small cell lung cancer. In: Pass HI, Carbone DP, Johnson DH, Minna JD, Scagliotti GV, Turrisi AT, eds. *Principles and Practice of Lung Cancer.* 4th ed. Philadelphia, PA: Lippincott Williams & Wilkins. 2010:521–529.

Quoix E, Ramlau R, Westeel V, Papai Z, Madroszyk A, Riviere A, Koralewski P, Breton JL, Stoelben E, Braun D, Debieuvre D, Lena H, Buyse M, Chenard MP, Acres B, Lacoste G, Bastien B, Tavernaro A, Bizouarne N, Bonnefoy JY, Limacher JM. Therapeutic vaccination with TG4010 and first-line chemotherapy in advanced non-small-cell lung cancer: a controlled phase 2B trial. *Lancet Oncol.* 2011;12(12):1125–1133. Epub 2011 Oct 21.

Schottenfeld D. The etiology and epidemiology of lung cancer. In: Pass HI, Carbone DP, Johnson DH, Minna JD, Scagliotti GV, Turrisi AT, eds. *Principles and Practice of Lung Cancer.* 4th ed. Philadelphia, PA: Lippincott Williams & Wilkins. 2010:3–22.

Schrump DS, Giaccone G, Kelsey CR, Marks LB. Non-small cell lung cancer. In: DeVita VT, Lawrence TS, Rosenberg SA, eds. *DeVita, Hellman, and Rosenberg's Cancer: Principles and Practice of Oncology.* 8th ed. Philadelphia, PA: Lippincott Williams & Wilkins; 2008:896–946.

Spigel DR, Townley PM, Waterhouse DM, Fang L, Adiguzel I, Huang JE, Karlin DA, Faoro L, Scappaticci FA, Socinski MA. Randomized phase II study of bevacizumab in combination with chemotherapy in previously untreated extensive-stage small-cell lung cancer: results from the SALUTE trial. *J Clin Oncol.* 2011;29(16):2215–2222. Epub 2011 Apr 18.

Travis WD, Brambilla E, Noguchi M, Nicholson AG, Geisinger KR, Yatabe Y, Beer DG, Powell CA, Riely GJ, Van Schil PE, Garg K, Austin JH, Asamura H, Rusch VW, Hirsch FR, Scagliotti G, Mitsudomi T, Huber RM, Ishikawa Y, Jett J, Sanchez-Cespedes M, Sculier JP, Takahashi T, Tsuboi M, Vansteenkiste J, Wistuba I, Yang PC, Aberle D, Brambilla C, Flieder D, Franklin W, Gazdar A, Gould M, Hasleton P, Henderson D, Johnson B, Johnson D, Kerr K, Kuriyama K, Lee JS, Miller VA, Petersen I, Roggli V, Rosell R, Saijo N, Thunnissen E, Tsao M, Yankelewitz D. International association for the study of lung cancer/american thoracic society/european respiratory society international multidisciplinary classification of lung adenocarcinoma. *J Thorac Oncol*. 2011;6(2):244–85.

U.S. Department of Health and Human Services. *The Health Consequences of Involuntary Exposure to Tobacco Smoke: A Report of the Surgeon General*. Washington, DC: Department of Health and Human Services; 2006. U.S. Department of Health and Human Services Web site. www.surgeongeneral.gov/library/secondhandsmoke. Accessed October 20, 2010.

U.S. Preventive Services Task Force. Lung cancer screening. *Ann Int Med*. 2004;140:738–739.

Wozniak AJ, Gadgeel SM. Clinical presentation of non-small cell carcinoma of the lung. In: Pass HI, Carbone DP, Johnson DH, Minna JD, Scagliotti GV, Turrisi AT, eds. *Principles and Practice of Lung Cancer*. 4th ed. Philadelphia, PA: Lippincott Williams & Wilkins. 2010:327–340.

Zhou W, Heist RS, Liu G, Asomaning K, Neuberg DS, Hollis BW, Wain JC, Lynch TJ, Giovannucci E, Su L, Christiani DC. Circulating 25-hydroxyvitamin D levels predict survival in early-stage non-small-cell lung cancer patients. *J Clin Oncol*. 2007;25(5):479–485.

Glossary

adenocarcinoma (add-uh-no-kahr-si-NO-muh): cancer that starts in the glandular tissue, such as in the ducts or lobules of the breast or the outer region of the lungs.

adjuvant therapy (AJ-uh-vunt therapy): treatment used in addition to the main treatment. It usually refers to hormonal therapy, chemotherapy, radiation therapy, or immunotherapy added after surgery to increase the chances of curing the disease or keeping it in check. *Compare with* neoadjuvant therapy.

alternative medicine: use of an unproven therapy instead of standard (proven) therapy. Some alternative therapies may have dangerous or even life-threatening side effects. With others, the main danger is that the patient may lose the opportunity to benefit from standard therapy. The American Cancer Society recommends that patients considering the use of any alternative or complementary therapies discuss them with their health care team. *Compare with* complementary medicine.

alveoli (al-VEE-o-lie): air sacs of the lungs.

American Joint Committee on Cancer (AJCC) staging system: a system for describing the extent of a cancer's spread by using Roman numerals from 0 through IV. Also called the TNM system. *See also* staging.

anesthesia (an-es-THEE-zhuh): the loss of feeling or sensation as a result of drugs or gases. **General anesthesia** causes loss of consciousness (makes you go into a deep sleep). **Local** or **regional anesthesia** numbs only a certain area of the body. **Epidural anesthesia** uses an injection of anesthetic drugs into the space around the spinal cord in order to numb the lower part of the body while allowing the patient to remain awake. *See also* anesthetic.

anesthetic: a topical or intravenous substance that causes loss of feeling or awareness in a part of the body. General anesthetics are used to put patients to sleep for procedures. *See also* anesthesia.

angiogenesis (an-jee-o-JEN-uh-sis): the formation of new blood vessels. Some cancer treatments work by blocking angiogenesis, thus preventing blood from reaching the tumor.

antibodies: proteins produced by the body's immune system cells and released into the blood. Antibodies defend the body against foreign agents, such as bacteria. These agents contain certain substances called antigens. Each antibody works against a specific antigen.

atypical (a-TIP-uh-kul): not usual; abnormal. Often refers to the appearance of cancerous or precancerous cells.

benign: not cancer; not malignant.

benign tumor: an abnormal growth that is not cancer and does not spread to other areas of the body.

biopsy (BUY-op-see): the removal of a sample of tissue to see whether cancer cells are present. There are several kinds of biopsies. In some, a very thin needle is used to draw fluid and cells from a lump. In a **core needle biopsy,** a larger needle is used to remove more tissue. *See also* CT–guided needle biopsy, transtracheal fine needle aspiration.

bone marrow aspiration: a procedure in which a small amount of bone marrow is removed for examination under a microscope. A small area of skin (usually over the hip bone, thigh bone, or breastbone) and the surface of the bone underneath are numbed with a local anesthetic. Then a needle is inserted into the bone and a small sample of liquid bone marrow is withdrawn.

bone marrow biopsy: a procedure in which a needle is placed into the cavity of a bone, usually the hip or breast bone, to remove a small amount of bone marrow for examination under a microscope.

bone scan: an imaging method that gives important information about the bones, including the location of cancer that may have spread to the bones. It can be done as an outpatient procedure and is painless, except for the needle stick when a low-dose radioactive substance is injected into a vein. Special pictures are taken to see where the radioactivity collects, pointing to an abnormality.

brachytherapy (brake-ee-THAYR-uh-pee): internal radiation treatment given by placing radioactive material directly into the tumor or close to it. Also called interstitial radiation therapy or seed implantation. *See* internal radiation. *Compare with* external beam radiation therapy.

bronchi (BRONG-ki): in the lungs, the 2 main air passages leading from the windpipe (trachea). The bronchi provide passages for air to move in and out of the lungs. The singular form of bronchi is bronchus.

bronchiole (BRONG-key-ol): one of the smaller sub-divisions of the bronchi.

bronchoscopy (brong-KOS-ko-pee): examination of the bronchi using a flexible, lighted tube called a bronchoscope.

cancer: cancer is not just one disease but a group of diseases. All forms of cancer cause cells in the body to change and grow out of control. Most types of cancer cells form a lump or mass called a tumor. The tumor can invade and destroy healthy tissue. Cells from the tumor can break away and travel to other parts of the body. There they can continue to grow. This spreading process is called metastasis. When cancer spreads, it is still named after the part of the body where it started. For example, if breast cancer spreads to the lungs, it is still called breast cancer, not lung cancer.

Some cancers, such as blood cancers, do not form a tumor. Not all tumors are cancer. A tumor that is not cancer is called benign. Benign tumors do not grow and spread the way cancer does. Benign tumors are usually not a threat to life. Another word for cancerous is malignant.

cancer care team: the group of health care professionals who work together to find, treat, and care for people with cancer. The cancer care team may include the following and others: primary care physicians, pathologists, oncology specialists (medical oncologist, radiation oncologist), surgeons (including surgical specialists such as urologists, gynecologists, neurosurgeons, etc.), nurses, oncology nurse specialists, and oncology social workers. Whether the team is linked formally or informally, there is usually one person who takes the job of coordinating the team.

carcinogen (kahr-SIN-o-jin): any substance that causes cancer or helps cancer grow. For example, tobacco smoke contains many carcinogens that greatly increase the risk of lung cancer.

carcinoid (KAHR-sih-noid) tumors or carcinoids: tumors that develop from neuroendocrine cells, usually in the digestive tract, lung, or ovary. The cancer cells from these tumors release certain hormones into the bloodstream. In about 10% of people, the hormone levels are high enough to cause facial flushing, wheezing, diarrhea, a fast heartbeat, and other symptoms throughout the body.

carcinoma (kahr-si-NO-muh): any cancerous tumor that begins in the lining layer of organs. At least 80% of all cancers are carcinomas.

carcinoma in situ (kahr-si-NO-muh in SIGH-too): an early stage of cancer in which the tumor is confined to the organ where it first developed. The disease has not invaded other parts of the organ or spread to distant parts of the body. Most in situ carcinomas are highly curable.

cell: the basic unit of which all living things are made. Cells replace themselves by splitting and forming new cells (mitosis). The processes that control the formation of new cells and the death of old cells are disrupted in cancer.

chemotherapy (key-mo-THAYR-uh-pee): treatment with drugs to destroy cancer cells. Chemotherapy is often used, either alone or with surgery or radiation, to treat cancer that has spread or come back (recurred), or when there is a strong chance that it could recur.

chromosome (KROM-o-some): chromosomes carry the genes, the basic units of heredity. Humans have 23 pairs of chromosomes, one member of each pair from the mother, the other from the father. Each chromosome can contain hundreds or thousands of individual genes. *See also* gene.

clinical stage: an estimate of the extent of cancer based on physical examination, biopsy results, and imaging tests. *See* staging. *Compare with* pathologic stage.

clinical trial: a research study to test new drugs or other treatments to compare current, standard treatments with others that may be better. Before a new treatment is used on people, it is studied in the laboratory. If laboratory studies suggest the treatment will work, the next step is to test its value for patients. These human studies are called clinical trials.

The main questions the researchers want to answer are these:

- Does this treatment work?
- Does it work better than what we're now using?
- What side effects does it cause?
- Do the benefits outweigh the risks?
- Which patients are most likely to find this treatment helpful?

complementary medicine: treatment used in addition to standard therapy. Some complementary therapies may help relieve certain symptoms of cancer, relieve side effects of standard cancer therapy, or improve a patient's sense of well-being. The American Cancer Society recommends that patients considering the use of any alternative or complementary therapies discuss these therapies with their cancer care team, since many of these treatments are unproven and some can be harmful. *Compare with* alternative medicine.

complete blood count (CBC): a test to check the level of red blood cells, white blood cells, and platelets in the blood.

computed tomography (to-MAHG-ruh-fee): an imaging test in which many x-rays are taken of a part of the body from different angles. These images are combined by a computer to produce cross-sectional pictures of internal organs. Except for the injection of a contrast dye (needed in some, but not all cases), this is a painless procedure that can be done in an outpatient clinic. It is often referred to as "CT" or "CAT" scanning.

contrast solution: any material used in imaging tests, such as x-rays and MRI and CT scans, to help outline the body parts being examined. These solutions may be injected or ingested (drunk). Also called contrast dye, radiocontrast dye, radiocontrast medium.

control group: in research or clinical trials, the group that does not receive the treatment being tested. The group may get a placebo or sham treatment, or it may receive standard therapy. Also called the comparison group. *See also* clinical trial.

core needle biopsy: *see* biopsy.

CT–guided needle biopsy: a procedure that uses special x-rays to locate a mass, while the radiologist advances a biopsy needle toward it. The images are repeated until the doctor is sure the needle is in the tumor or mass. A small sample of tissue is then taken from the mass to be examined under a microscope. *See also* biopsy.

CT scan or CAT scan: *see* computed tomography.

deoxyribonucleic acid (dee-ok-see-ri-bo-new-CLAY-ic acid): the genetic "blueprint" found in the nucleus of each cell. DNA holds genetic information on cell growth, division, and function.

diagnosis: identifying a disease by its signs or symptoms and by using imaging procedures and laboratory findings. For some types of cancer, the earlier a diagnosis is made, the better the chance for long-term survival.

diaphragm: the thin muscle that separates the chest from the abdomen.

DNA: *see* deoxyribonucleic acid.

DNA repair: the process of correcting the genetic mistakes that are made each time a cell divides. If there are mistakes during the repair process, it can increase the chances of a person having some forms of cancer. *See also* deoxyribonucleic acid.

endobronchial ultrasound: a test used to examine lymph nodes and other structures in the mediastinum. The patient is given a local anesthetic and a sedative, and a bronchoscope is passed down the trachea to examine these areas.

endoscopic esophageal ultrasound (en-do-SKOP-ik uh-sof-uh-JEE-uhl ultrasound) (EUS): a method in which a lighted, flexible scope is passed through the esophagus to permit ultrasound imaging from inside the esophagus. This method is useful for detecting large lymph nodes in the chest that may contain metastatic cancer.

epidermal growth factor receptor (EGFR): a protein found on the surface of some cells. Epidermal growth factor binds to EGFR and causes the cells to divide. EGFR is found in high levels on the surface of many cancer cells.

extensive stage: a term used to describe the extent of small cell lung cancer. Extensive stage describes cancers that have spread to the other lung, to lymph nodes on the other side of the chest, or to distant organs. *Compare with* limited stage.

external beam radiation therapy (EBRT): radiation that is focused from a source outside the body on the area affected by the cancer. It is much like getting a diagnostic x-ray, but for a longer period. *See also* radiation therapy. *Compare with* brachytherapy.

fatigue (fuh-TEEG): a common symptom during cancer treatment, a bone-weary exhaustion that doesn't get better with rest. For some, this condition can last for some time after treatment.

FDA: *see* U.S. Food and Drug Administration.

fine needle aspiration (FNA) biopsy: a procedure in which a thin needle is used to draw up (aspirate) samples for examination under a microscope. *See also* biopsy, needle biopsy.

five (5)-year survival rate: the percentage of people with a given cancer who are expected to survive 5 years or longer with the disease. Five-year survival rates have some drawbacks. Although the rates are based on the most recent information available, they may include data from patients treated several years earlier. Advances in cancer treatment often occur quickly. Five-year survival rates, while statistically valid, may not reflect these advances. They should not be seen as a predictor in any individual case. *Compare with* relative five (5)-year survival rate.

fluorescence bronchoscopy: a procedure in which a bronchoscope, a long thin tube, is inserted into the mouth and through the windpipe into the lung. The bronchoscope contains a light and eyepiece that allows the doctor to look into the airways of the lung. The fluorescent light helps to detect lung cancers in early stages.

gene: a segment of DNA that contains information on hereditary characteristics such as hair color, eye color, and height, as well as susceptibility to certain diseases. *See also* DNA.

grade: the grade of a cancer reflects how abnormal it looks under the microscope. There are several grading systems for different types of cancer. Each grading system divides cancer into those with the greatest abnormality, the least abnormality, and those in between.

Grading is done by a pathologist who examines the tissue from the biopsy. The grade of the cancer is important because cancers with more abnormal-appearing cells tend to grow and spread more quickly and have a worse prognosis (outlook).

Hodgkin disease (HOJ-kin dih-ZEEZ): a cancer of the immune system that is marked by the presence of a type of cell called the Reed-Sternberg cell. The two major types of Hodgkin disease are classical Hodgkin lymphoma and nodular lymphocyte–predominant Hodgkin lymphoma. Symptoms include the painless enlargement of lymph nodes, spleen, or other immune system tissue. Other symptoms include fever, weight loss, fatigue, or night sweats. Also called Hodgkin lymphoma.

hospice: a special kind of care for people in the final phase of illness, their families, and caregivers. The care may take place in the patient's home or in a home-like facility.

hypercalcemia (hy-per-kal-SEE-mee-uh): a high calcium level in the blood, sometimes due to cancer cells causing the release of calcium from bones.

imaging tests: methods used to produce pictures of internal body structures. Some imaging methods used to help diagnose or stage cancer are x-rays, CT scans, magnetic resonance imaging (MRI), and ultrasound.

immune system: the complex system by which the body resists infection by germs such as bacteria or viruses and rejects transplanted tissues or organs. The immune system may also help the body fight some cancers.

informed consent: a legal document that explains a course of treatment, the risks, benefits, and possible alternatives; the process by which patients agree to treatment.

internal radiation: treatment involving implantation of a radioactive substance. *See* brachytherapy. *Compare with* external beam radiation therapy.

large-cell undifferentiated carcinoma: cancer that may appear in any part of the lung. The cells are large and look abnormal when viewed under a microscope. They tend to grow and spread quickly.

laser therapy: treatment that uses intense, narrow beams of light to cut and destroy cancer tissue.

limited stage: a term used to describe the extent of small cell lung cancer. Limited stage typically means that the cancer is confined to one lung and perhaps lymph nodes on the same side of the chest. *Compare with* extensive stage.

lobe: a well-defined portion of an organ such as the brain, lung, liver, breast, or gland.

lobectomy (lob-BEK-to-me): surgery to remove a lobe of an organ—usually the lung.

lymph (limf): clear fluid that flows through the lymphatic vessels and contains cells known as lymphocytes. These cells are important in fighting infections and may also have a role in fighting cancer. *See also* lymphatic system, lymph nodes.

lymphatic system: a network of tissues and organs (including lymph nodes, spleen, thymus, and bone marrow) that produce and store lymphocytes (cells that fight infection) and the channels that carry the lymph fluid. The lymphatic system is an important part of the body's immune system, as its function is to fight infection. Invasive cancers sometimes penetrate the lymphatic vessels (channels) and spread (metastasize) to lymph nodes. *See also* lymph, lymph nodes.

lymph nodes: small bean-shaped collections of immune system tissue such as lymphocytes that are found along lymphatic vessels. They remove cell waste, germs, and other harmful substances from lymph. They help fight infections and also have a role in fighting cancer, although cancers sometimes spread through lymph nodes. Also called lymph glands. *See also* lymph, lymphatic system.

magnetic resonance imaging (MRI): a method of taking pictures of the inside of the body. Instead of using x-rays, MRI uses a powerful magnet to send radio waves through the body. The images appear on a computer screen, as well as on film. Like x-rays, the procedure is physically painless, but some people may feel confined inside the MRI machine.

malignant: cancerous.

mediastinoscopy (me-dee-uh-stine-AHS-ko-pee): examination of the chest cavity using a lighted tube inserted under the chest bone (sternum). This allows the doctor to examine the lymph nodes in this area and remove samples to check for cancer. *See also* mediastinum.

mediastinotomy (me-dee-uh-stine-AH-to-mee): a procedure in which the doctor makes an incision into the mediastinum. *See also* mediastinum, mediastinoscopy.

mediastinum (me-dee-uh-STI-nuhm): the space in the chest cavity behind the chest bone (sternum) and between the 2 lungs.

mesothelioma: a benign or malignant tumor, typically found in the lining of the chest or abdomen. Malignant mesothelioma is related to exposure to asbestos.

metastasis (meh-TAS-teh-sis): cancer cells that have spread to one or more sites elsewhere in the body, often by way of the lymphatic system or bloodstream. **Regional metastasis** is cancer that has spread to the lymph nodes, tissues, or organs close to the primary site. **Distant metastasis** is cancer that has spread to organs or tissues that are farther away (such as when lung cancer spreads to the brain). The plural of this word is metastases.

metastasize (meh-TAS-tuh-size): the spread of cancer cells to one or more sites elsewhere in the body, often by way of the lymphatic system or bloodstream.

metastatic (met-uh-STAT-ick) cancer: a way to describe cancer that has spread from the primary site (where it started) to other structures or organs, nearby or far away (distant).

monoclonal (ma-nuh-KLO-nuhl) antibody: a type of antibody manufactured in the laboratory. Monoclonal antibodies are designed to lock onto specific antigens (substances that can be recognized by the immune system). Monoclonal antibodies that have been attached to chemotherapy drugs or radioactive substances are being studied for their potential to seek out antigens unique to cancer cells and go directly to the cancer, thus killing the cancer cells and not harming healthy tissue. Monoclonal antibodies are also often used to help detect and classify cancer cells under a microscope. Other studies are being done to determine whether radioactive atoms attached to monoclonal antibodies can be used in imaging tests to detect and locate small groups of cancer cells. *See also* antibodies.

MRI: *see* magnetic resonance imaging.

mutation (myoo-TAY-shun): a change in the DNA of a cell. Most mutations do not produce cancer, and a few may even be helpful. However, all types of cancer are thought to be due to mutations that damage a cell's DNA. Some cancer-related mutations can be inherited, which means that the person is born with the mutated DNA in all the body's cells. But most mutations happen after the person is born, and are called somatic mutations. This type of mutation happens in one cell at a time and only affects cells that arise from the single mutated cell. *See also* DNA, gene.

neoadjuvant (nee-oh-AJ-oo-vunt) therapy: treatment given before the main treatment. *Compare with* adjuvant therapy.

non–small cell lung cancer: the most common kind of lung cancer. This group of cancers is named for the kinds of cells found and how they appear under a microscope. The main types of non–small cell lung cancer are squamous cell carcinoma, adenocarcinoma, and large-cell undifferentiated carcinoma.

oncogenes: genes that promote cell growth and multiplication. These genes are normally present in all cells. But oncogenes may undergo changes that activate them, causing cells to grow too quickly and form tumors.

palliative (PAL-ee-uh-tiv) care: treatment that relieves symptoms, such as pain or blockage of urine flow, but is not expected to cure the disease. Its main purpose is to improve the patient's quality of life. Sometimes chemotherapy and radiation are used as palliative treatments.

paraneoplastic syndromes: a group of symptoms that can develop when substances released by cancer cells disrupt the normal function of surrounding cells and tissues.

pathologic stage: an estimate of the extent of cancer by direct study of the samples removed during surgery. *See* staging. *Compare with* clinical stage.

PET scan: *see* positron emission tomography.

photodynamic therapy (foe-toe-die-NAM-ick therapy) (PDT): a treatment sometimes used for cancers of the skin, esophagus, lung, or bladder. PDT begins with the injection of a nontoxic chemical into the blood. This chemical is attracted to cancer cells and is allowed to collect in the tumor for a few days. A special type of laser light is then focused on the cancer. This light causes the chemical to change so that it can kill cancer cells. The advantage of PDT is that it can kill cancer cells with very little harm to healthy tissues.

pleura (PLOO-ruh): the membrane around the lungs and lining of the chest cavity.

pleural effusion: a collection of fluid between the chest wall and the pleura, the thin layers of tissue lining the lungs.

pleurodesis (ploo-row-DEE-sis): injection of an agent between the layers of the pleura that causes them to fuse together to seal off leaks. This procedure helps prevent fluid or air from building up in the pleural cavity. *See also* pleura.

pneumonectomy (new-mo-NEK-to-me): surgery to remove an entire lung.

positron emission tomography (PAHS-ih-trahn ee-MISH-uhn toh-MAHG-ruh-fee) (PET): a PET scan creates an image of the body (or of biochemical events) after the injection of a very low dose of a radioactive form of a substance such as glucose (sugar). The scan computes the rate at which the tumor is using the sugar. In general, high-grade tumors use more sugar than normal and low-grade tumors use less. PET scans are especially useful in taking images of the brain, although they are becoming more widely used to find the spread of cancer of the breast, colon, rectum, ovary, or lung. PET scans may also be used to see how well the tumor is responding to treatment.

precancerous: changes in cells that may, but do not always, become cancer.

primary site: the place where cancer begins. Primary cancer is usually named after the organ in which it starts. For example, cancer that starts in the breast is always breast cancer even if it spreads (metastasizes) to other organs such as bones or lungs.

prognosis (prog-NO-sis): a prediction of the course of disease; the outlook for the chances of survival.

pulmonary function tests (PFTs): tests to measure how well the lungs are working. Pulmonary function tests can measure how much air the person's lungs can hold and how quickly air can be moved in and out of the lungs.

radiation therapy (RAY-dee-AY-shun THAYR-un-pee): treatment with high-energy rays (such as x-rays) to kill or shrink cancer cells. The radiation may come from outside of the body (external radiation) or from radioactive materials placed directly in the tumor (brachytherapy or internal radiation). Radiation therapy may be used as the main treatment for a cancer, to reduce the size of a cancer before surgery, or to destroy any remaining cancer cells after surgery. In advanced cancer cases, it may also be used as palliative treatment. *See also* brachytherapy, internal radiation, external beam radiation therapy.

radiofrequency ablation (RAY-dee-oh-free-kwin-see uh-BLAY-shun): treatment that uses electric current to destroy abnormal tissues. A thin, needle-like probe is guided into the tumor by ultrasound or CT scan. The probe releases a high-frequency current that heats and destroys cancer cells.

randomized or randomization: a process used in clinical trials that uses chance to assign participants to different groups that compare treatments. Randomization means that each person has an equal chance of being in the treatment and comparison groups. This helps reduce the chance of bias in the results that might happen, if, for example, the healthiest people all were assigned to a particular treatment group. *See also* clinical trial, control group.

recurrence: the return of cancer after treatment. **Local recurrence** means that the cancer has come back at the same place as the original cancer. **Regional recurrence** means that the cancer has come back after treatment in the lymph nodes near the primary site. **Distant recurrence**, also known as metastatic recurrence, is when cancer metastasizes *after* treatment to distant organs or tissues (such as the liver, bone marrow, or brain).

relative five (5)-year survival rate: the percentage of people with a specific cancer who have not died of it within 5 years. This number is different from the 5-year survival rate in that it does not include people who have died of unrelated causes. *Compare with* five (5)-year survival rate.

remission: complete or partial disappearance of the signs and symptoms of cancer in response to treatment; the period during which a disease is under control. A remission may not be a cure.

risk factor: anything that affects a person's chance of getting a disease such as cancer. Different cancers have different risk factors. For example, unprotected exposure to strong sunlight is a risk factor for skin cancer; smoking is a risk factor for lung, mouth, larynx, and other cancers. Some risk factors, such as smoking, can be controlled. Others, like a person's age, can't be changed.

screening: the search for disease, such as cancer, in people without symptoms. For example, screening measures for prostate cancer include digital rectal examination and the prostate-specific antigen (PSA) blood test. Screening may refer to coordinated programs in large populations.

secondhand smoke: smoke that comes from the burning of tobacco products and the exhaled smoke of smokers. Also called environmental tobacco smoke.

segmentectomy: removal of part of a lobe (section) of the lung. Also known as wedge resection.

side effects: unwanted effects of treatment, such as hair loss caused by chemotherapy and fatigue caused by radiation therapy.

sign: an observable physical change caused by an illness. *Compare with* symptom.

sleeve resection: surgery in which a tumor in a lobe of the lung and a part of the main bronchus (airway) is removed. The ends of the bronchus are rejoined and any remaining lobes are reattached to the bronchus. This surgery is done to save part of the lung.

small cell lung cancer: an aggressive (fast-growing) kind of cancer that forms in the tissues of the lung and can spread to other parts of the body. Other names for small cell lung cancer are oat cell cancer, oat cell carcinoma, and small cell undifferentiated carcinoma.

spiral CT: a special scanner that takes cross-sectional pictures around the body. Also called helical CT. *See also* computed tomography.

sputum cytology (SPU-tum sigh-TAHL-uh-gee): a study of phlegm cells under a microscope to see whether they are normal or not.

squamous cell carcinoma (SKWAY-mus cell kahr-si-NO-muh): cancer that begins in the non-glandular cells, for example, the skin.

stage: the extent of a cancer in the body. *See* staging.

staging: the process of finding out whether cancer has spread and if so, how far. The AJCC/TNM system gives 3 key pieces of information:
- T refers to the size of the tumor
- N describes how far the cancer has spread to nearby lymph nodes
- M shows whether the cancer has spread (metastasized) to other organs of the body

Letters or numbers after the T, N, and M give more details about each of these factors. To make this information more clear, the TNM descriptions can be grouped together into a simpler set of stages, labeled with Roman numerals (usually from I to IV). In general, the lower the number, the less the cancer has spread. A higher number means a more serious cancer.

The 2 types of staging are clinical staging and pathologic staging.

stereotactic body radiation therapy (SBRT): a type of external radiation therapy that uses special equipment to precisely position the patient and deliver radiation to tumors in the body. The total amount of radiation is divided into smaller doses given over the course of several days. This type of radiation therapy is less damaging to healthy tissues. *See also* external beam radiation therapy.

symptom: a change in the body caused by an illness, as described by the person experiencing it. *Compare with* sign.

targeted therapies: treatments that attack the part of cancer cells that makes them different from normal cells, as opposed to treatment that harms all cells. Targeted therapy tends to have fewer side effects than some standard treatments such as chemotherapy.

thoracentesis (thor-uh-sen-TEE-sis): a procedure during which the skin is numbed and a needle is placed between the ribs to drain fluid that surrounds the lung. The fluid is checked under a microscope to look for cancer cells. Fluid buildup can prevent the lungs from filling with air, so thoracentesis can help the patient breathe more easily and may be repeated as needed.

thoracoscopy (thor-uh-KAH-skuh-pee): a procedure during which small incisions are made in the chest to permit insertion of surgical tools such as the thorascope—a long tube with a magnifying glass and light on the end. This procedure permits the doctor to see suspicious areas and remove tissues to be examined.

thoracotomy: an operation to open the chest.

tissue: a collection of cells, united to perform a particular function in the body.

TNM staging system: *see* staging.

TP53: an important tumor suppressor gene that is not working properly in many cancers. The protein that this gene makes (also called p53) normally causes damaged cells to die. Mutations, or changes, in this gene can be inherited or they can occur during a person's life. When they do occur, they can increase risk of getting many types of cancer. *See also* mutation, tumor suppressor gene.

trachea (TRAY-key-uh): the "windpipe." The trachea connects the larynx (voice box) with the bronchi and serves as the main passage for air into the lungs.

transtracheal fine needle aspiration (trans-TRAY-kee-uhl fine needle aspiration): a procedure by which a thin needle is inserted into the wall of the trachea and guided by bronchoscopy to sample nearby lymph nodes. This method is used to detect cancerous cells and determine whether cancer has spread.

tumor: an abnormal lump or mass of tissue. Tumors can be benign (noncancerous) or malignant (cancerous).

tumor suppressor genes: genes that slow down cell division or cause cells to die at the appropriate time. Alterations of these genes can lead to too much cell growth and the development of cancer.

ultrasound: an imaging method in which high-frequency sound waves are used to outline a part of the body. The sound wave echoes are picked up and displayed on a television screen. Also called ultrasonography.

U.S. Food and Drug Administration (FDA): an agency of the United States Department of Health and Human Services. The FDA is responsible for regulating drugs, tobacco products, biological medical products, blood products, medical devices, and radiation-emitting devices, along with other products.

video-assisted thoracic surgery (VATS): a type of thoracic surgery that is performed by using a small video camera, which allows doctors to see the inside of the chest cavity after making only small incisions. VATS is less invasive than a thoracotomy.

virtual bronchoscopy: a noninvasive procedure that uses computed tomography to create 3-dimensional images of the airways in the lungs. It allows doctors to see airways that may not be visible with standard bronchoscopy.

wedge resection: surgery to remove a triangle-shaped slice of tissue. It may be used to remove a tumor and a small amount of normal tissue around it.

x-ray: one form of radiation that can be used at low levels to produce an image of the body on film or at high levels to destroy cancer cells.

Index

Books Published
by the American Cancer Society

Information

The American Cancer Society: A History of Saving Lives

American Cancer Society Complete Guide to Complementary and Alternative Cancer Therapies, Second Edition

American Cancer Society Complete Guide to Nutrition for Cancer Survivors, Second Edition

QuickFACTS™ Advanced Cancer

QuickFACTS™ Bone Metastasis

Day-to-Day Help

American Cancer Society Complete Guide to Family Caregiving, Second Edition

Kicking Butts: Quit Smoking and Take Charge of Your Health, Second Edition

Lymphedema: Understanding and Managing Lymphedema After Cancer Treatment

What to Eat During Cancer Treatment: 100 Great-Tasting, Family-Friendly Recipes to Help You Cope

Emotional Support

And Still They Bloom: A Family's Journey of Loss and Healing

Couples Confronting Cancer: Keeping Your Relationship Strong

I Can Survive

Picture Your Life After Cancer

Rad Art: A Journey Through Radiation Treatment

The Survivorship Net: A Parable for the Family, Friends, and Caregivers of People with Cancer

What Helped Get Me Through: Cancer Survivors Share Wisdom and Hope

Just For Kids

Because . . . Someone I Love Has Cancer

Healthy Me: A Read-Along Coloring & Activity Book

Let My Colors Out

The Long and the Short of It: A Tale About Hair

Nana, What's Cancer?

No Thanks, but I'd Love to Dance: Choosing to Live Smoke Free

Our Dad Is Getting Better

Our Mom Has Cancer (available in hard cover and paperback)

Our Mom Is Getting Better

Prevention

The American Cancer Society's Healthy Eating Cookbook: A Celebration of Food, Friends, and Healthy Living, Third Edition

The Great American Eat-Right Cookbook

Healthy Air: A Read-Along Coloring and Activity Book (25 per pack: Tobacco avoidance)

For a complete listing of books published by the American Cancer Society, go to the Web site:
www.cancer.org/bookstore